MW01280307

HORMONES
MOLECULAR
MESSENGERS

JOHN K. YOUNG

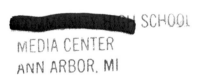
A Venture Book
Franklin Watts
New York/Chicago/London/Toronto/Sydney

Photographs copyright ©: Photo Researchers, Inc.: p. 51; UPI/Bettmann
Newsphotos: p. 64; all other photographs courtesy of the author.

Library of Congress Cataloging-in-Publication Data

Young, John K.
Hormones : molecular messengers / by John K. Young.
p.   cm.—(A Venture book.)
Includes bibliographical references and index.
Summary: Provides an introduction to the endocrine system,
focusing on the human body's major hormones and the organs affected
by them.
ISBN 0-531-12545-9
1. Hormones—Juvenile literature.   2. Endocrinology—Juvenile
literature.   [1. Hormones.   2. Endocrine glands.]   I. Title.
QP571.Y68   1993
612.4—dc20   92-40503   CIP   AC

CONTENTS

ENDOCRINOLOGY:
A BRIEF
INTRODUCTION

My first exposure to hormones—or at any rate, my first exposure in a scientific setting—came about when I was a junior in college. I was working in a lab and was asked to weigh out a small quantity of thyroid hormone. I dutifully got out a little bottle and poured out some dried, fluffy crystals of thyroid hormone onto a piece of weighing paper. Because I had shaken the bottle too much, a few tiny motes flew up into the air and drifted around like particles of dust. My instructor immediately turned to me and admonished: "You'd better be more careful with that, John; if you breathe in a few of those you'll be climbing the walls all night!"

My instructor's concern about the potency and hazard of those few tiny crystals of hormone may have been a bit misplaced—while thyroid hormone is powerful, it is not quite the pixie dust of fairy tales that can magically transform a person in a twinkling. Nevertheless, hormones have enough similarity to magical substances to make them truly fascinating as well as valuable to understand from a medical standpoint. Hormones are extremely powerful and can exert drastic effects upon many organ systems of the body in very small doses. Many other substances that affect our health, such as nutrients and vitamins, are powerful in their own right: as little as a gram of some nutrients—as much as a kernel of corn would weigh—can have important effects upon health, and vitamins can be given effectively in doses as little as one thousandth of a gram (a milligram). Hormones, however, can have dramatic effects upon our bodies in doses as small as a millionth of a gram (a microgram). This is possible because certain cells in the body are constructed to respond to even a few dozen molecules of a hormone at a time with greatly amplified changes in cell function. In this book, I would like to introduce you to some of the many fascinating hormones that transform our bodies throughout our lives and to explain what these hormones accomplish.

WHAT ARE HORMONES?

The definition of a **hormone** is simple: anything that is produced by one organ and then carried via the bloodstream to another organ—called a "target organ"—and that affects the second organ's function. Most organs that produce hormones are glands, and since they secrete something into the bloodstream they are called **endocrine glands**, after the Greek words for "secrete within" (see Figure 1). The other type of glands in the body secrete something into ducts connected to hollow organs, such as the ducts of the salivary glands. Since these ducts lead into hollow organs such as the mouth that are in communication with the outside world, the glands using ducts for secretion are called "exocrine glands," from the Greek for "secrete outside."

In previous years, it used to be just as simple a task to

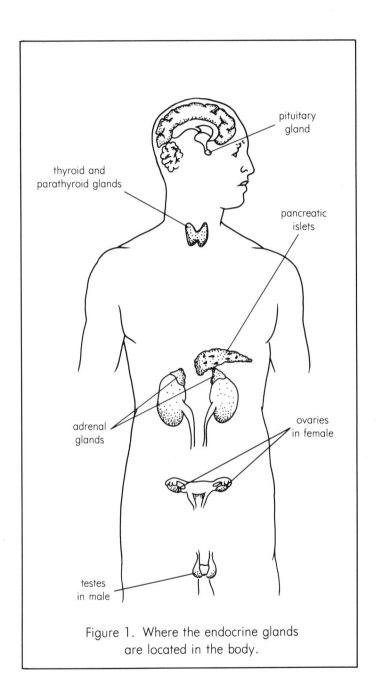

pituitary
gland

thyroid and
parathyroid glands

pancreatic
islets

adrenal
glands

ovaries
in female

testes
in male

Figure 1. Where the endocrine glands
are located in the body.

list the known hormones as it was to give the definition of hormones. At most, seven endocrine organs were known, all producing a small quantity of hormones. Since these early years in the study of hormones, or endocrinology, the picture has gotten much more complicated. An astonishing variety of organs in the body are now known to produce their own hormones. The kidney, for example, produces hormones that affect blood pressure and blood cell development. The intestines produce hormones that affect digestion. The thymus gland is now known not only to produce cells of the immune system, but also hormones that affect their function as they migrate around the body. Even the heart is now known to be an endocrine organ, producing a hormone called atrial natriuretic peptide that affects blood pressure.

This new knowledge presents us with a real dilemma. How can a brief book even begin to talk about all the hormones that are known to exist? What should be left in and what should be left out? So many hormones are now known that the real question of endocrinology is not which organs make hormones, but rather which organs *do not* make them. Fortunately, there is a way out for us; namely, we can for the time being ignore hormones produced by organs that have other, nonendocrine tasks to fulfill. For example, in addition to making hormones, the heart pumps blood around the body and the intestines digest our food. By paying attention to only the classical endocrine organs, which make hormones and do nothing else, we can do justice to a selected portion of what is now understood as the endocrine system.

O N E

INSULIN

INSULIN AND DIABETES MELLITUS

One of the earliest hormones to be discovered was **insulin**. We now know that insulin is produced by certain cells located in a digestive gland called the **pancreas**. This gland is rather difficult to locate and amounts to a pinkish-gray collection of delicate glandular tissue suspended among sheets of fat and connective tissue attached to the small intestine, stomach, and spleen. For a long time the pancreas was regarded as simply an organ that manufactures digestive juices (**enzymes**) and squirts them into the intestine through a duct to help digest food. This, indeed, is an important function of the pancreas. Its role as an endocrine organ was only gradually understood as it became clear that the pancreas is involved in a devastating disease called **diabetes mellitus** (die-uh-BEET-ees MEL-ut-us).

Diabetes mellitus has been known since antiquity—

ancient Chinese and Egyptian manuscripts have been found that describe its major symptoms quite accurately. The most obvious symptom of the disease is excessive urination ("diabetes" is Greek for "to pass through") and an accompanying excessive thirst. Diabetes used to be regarded with almost the same dread as **cancer** now is: afflicted patients gradually wasted away and died. Aside from special diets that tended to slow this process, little could be done to help, since the cause and cure for diabetes were unknown. Then, almost by accident, a link between diabetes and the pancreas became known.

In 1889 a team of physiologists, J. von Mering and Oscar Minkowski in Strasbourg, removed the pancreas from dogs to see what effect this would have upon the digestion of food. To their surprise, the dogs remained able to digest their food to some extent but soon developed severe diabetes and died.

This caused a flurry of excitement and renewed interest in the pancreas. The French physiologist G. E. Laguesse recalled reading an obscure report on the pancreas written by a young German medical student named Paul Langerhans in 1869. Langerhans, in his graduation thesis, had found previously unknown collections of **cells** scattered throughout the pancreas; while their function remained unknown to Langerhans (he died in 1883), Laguesse suspected their importance in diabetes and named them the **islets** (EYE-lets—"little islands") **of Langerhans** in their discoverer's honor.

The involvement of these islet cells in diabetes was soon confirmed by Eugene Opie at Johns Hopkins University, who found that infectious damage to the islets could cause diabetes, and that many diabetics proved to have peculiar accumulations of shapeless material called "amyloid" in their islets. A view of a pancreatic islet, surrounded on all sides by darker-staining exocrine cells that produce pancreatic digestive juices and deliver them to the intestine through ducts, is shown in Figure 2. Soon

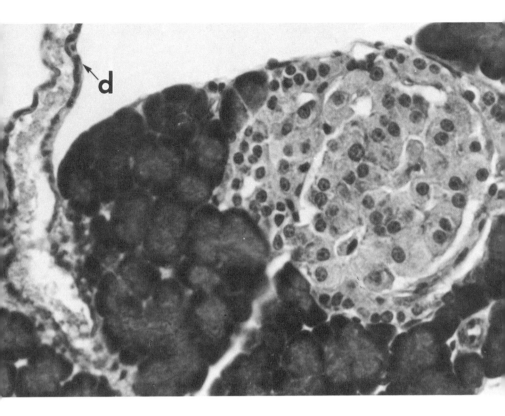

Figure 2. A pale-staining islet of Langerhans, surrounded by dark-staining cells of the pancreas that produce digestive enzymes. A small duct (d) that carries these enzymes to the intestine is also shown.

the race was on to discover how these islet cells could be involved in this disease.

Although many people were involved in this quest, the team most often credited with success was that of Frederick Banting and Charles Best, two physiologists working in Toronto in the laboratory of their professor, Dr. J. J. R. MacLeod. In 1921, Banting and Best decided they would try to separate out islets from the pancreas by a new approach: by tying off the main duct of the pancreas, they hoped that digestive juices would accumulate, digest and destroy most pancreatic tissue, and leave little behind except the islets. Amazingly, this approach worked—at any rate, if this process of self-digestion didn't proceed too far—and Banting and Best were able to gather together large amounts of relatively pure batches of islet cells. By grinding up these cells and making chemical extracts, they were able to isolate a substance that cured diabetes in dogs. They named this substance "insulin." It was not long before insulin was being used to treat people with diabetes mellitus.

The medical importance of this discovery was so great that Banting and MacLeod were awarded the Nobel Prize in 1923. One sad part of this story was that Banting's work, as he freely acknowledged, was partly based on published research by a Rumanian physiologist, Nicolas Paulesco, who had done experiments very similar to Banting and Best's. The Nobel committee failed to recognize Paulesco's contribution, so that he never got the recognition he deserved. This is not the first or only example of unfairness that can be encountered in science, or indeed, in many endeavors. Paulesco could at least take consolation from the fact that he had helped create new and valuable knowledge that would still be helping people long after even awards and honors like the Nobel Prize have become dim memories in dusty textbooks.

These discoveries were the start of many experiments that have clarified how insulin is involved in diabetes and in the control of metabolism. Many of these experiments have used special chemicals that can injure islet cells in, for example, laboratory rats so that the effects of insulin deficiency can be studied. A lack of insulin in an animal has dramatic effects: a rat will begin to drink (and urinate) much larger volumes of fluid, as much as five times the normal amount. Food intake may also double, but in spite of this, the rat will steadily lose weight unless therapeutic doses of insulin are given. Why do these things happen?

SYMPTOMS AND TREATMENT OF DIABETES MELLITUS

All of these effects result from a fundamental action of insulin: insulin, carried away from the islets through the bloodstream, stimulates muscle cells and fat cells to take up sugar (**glucose**) from the blood and metabolize (burn or store) it. Without insulin, cells cannot take up glucose, so it accumulates in the bloodstream to reach three to four times the normal level. This elevated level of blood sugar leads to a number of effects that can harm a diabetic's health.

One problem in diabetes is that diabetics cannot regulate the amount of water in the body as well as normal people. There are several reasons for this. First, a high concentration of glucose in the blood tends to cause water to leave cells. This is due to a physical property called **osmosis** (oz-MO-sis), according to which water will always flow from a dilute solution of sugar into a more concentrated solution of sugar if the two solutions are separated from each other by a porous membrane that lets water, but not other molecules, pass through. Osmosis is nature's way of attempting to make the concentrations of sugar in two different solutions equal; in diabetics, it causes water in cells to flow out through the membrane surrounding them and into the more concentrated solution of sugar in the bloodstream.

All this water eventually reaches the kidneys, which filter the blood to remove wastes. The kidneys cannot prevent high levels of glucose from passing into the urine. Loss of all this water and sugar in the urine is the reason why diabetic people, and diabetic rats, drink and eat so much but still lose weight. Also, high levels of blood glucose tend to damage structures in the kidney that filter the blood, so that diabetics may eventually have abnormal kidney function.

What can be done to help diabetics? Moderate, regular exercise is one thing that seems to help, since exercise somehow makes muscles more sensitive to insulin and allows them to remove some of the glucose from the blood. Once in a while, exercise can actually make muscles *too* sensitive to insulin, so that too much glucose is removed from the blood, making a diabetic feel sick or faint. This is why diabetics can eat sweets in these occasional emergency situations when their blood sugar actually falls too low. Eating the sweets raises their blood sugar and makes them feel better.

Eating regularly spaced, moderate meals is also helpful in preventing blood sugar in diabetics from becoming too high or too low. Also, drugs (called sulphonylureas— sul-fon-eel-you-REE-as) can be taken to stimulate the secretion of insulin by the pancreas. Finally, injections of insulin can be used to regulate blood sugar. Nowadays, specially modified forms of insulin are available that are slowly absorbed from the injection site and act for a long time, allowing a minimal number of injections per day. More recent advances involve miniature insulin pumps that introduce a steady flow of insulin into the bloodstream.

INSULIN AND THE CONTROL OF APPETITE

One question that has long puzzled scientists studying insulin is how a diabetic rat "knows" that it should eat and drink so much to make up for loss of nutrients in the urine. The basis for this behavioral reaction is an effect of insulin that is now recognized as a general property of many hormones: in addition to affecting the function of the body, insulin can also affect the function of the brain.

14

Figure 3 shows a series of cross sections through the brain of a mouse, photographed through the microscope at an increasing series of magnifications. The top panel shows the brain as a whole: its upper surface is known as the cortex, which is generally responsible for the thinking and planning that are part of the life of even a mouse. Below the cortex are a large number of complex structures that form and store memories and perform other functions: at the very bottom of the brain is the **hypothalamus** (hy-po-THAL-a-mus).

The hypothalamus, illustrated at a greater magnification in the middle panel of Figure 3, is of great importance in understanding the endocrine system: it controls and in turn is controlled by hormones.

Each tiny, dark dot visible in Figure 3 represents a single nerve cell. It is easy to see from this that the hypothalamus is made up of millions of nerve cells. Some of these are gathered into cell-dense accumulations called hypothalamic nuclei. Two of these nuclei, present in two copies on each side of the midline of the brain, are identified by numbers in Figure 3. One of these nuclei, the arcuate nucleus, is an important site of action of insulin.

When an animal becomes diabetic, it starts to overeat dramatically to try to recover all the calories lost as sugar in the urine, as we have said. What, however, causes this? Work in the lab of J. D. White at the State University of New York at Stony Brook has recently provided part of the answer to this question. White and others have examined special nerve cells in the arcuate nucleus of the hypothalamus that contain a certain chemical called neuropeptide Y. Neuropeptide Y, when infused into the brain of a rat, is the strongest stimulator of feeding known and can affect behavior in doses as small as a *billionth* of a gram! Normally, the nerve cells containing this chemical are not very active. When insulin levels in the blood fall, however, these cells explode into activity and start sending their chemical into parts of the brain that regulate swal-

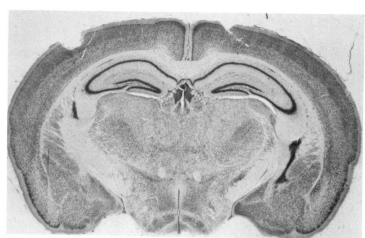

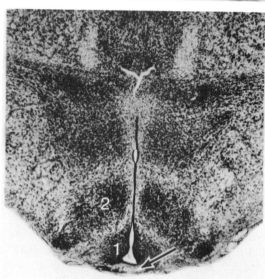

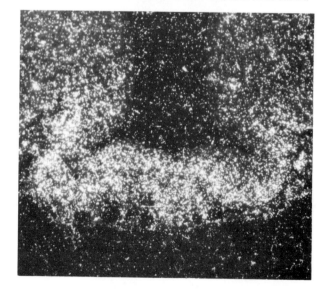

lowing, salivation, stomach activity, etc., so that the rat promptly feels hungry and starts eating like crazy.

Once again, how does the hypothalamus "know" that insulin levels in the blood have fallen? This question is not as simply answered as you would think, because normally most parts of the brain are supplied by special sealed blood vessels that protect the brain from blood-borne poisons or other harmful things. Most parts of the brain, in fact, are not exposed to insulin, which cannot pass through the blood vessel walls that constitute the so-called **blood-brain barrier**. The hypothalamus, however, is next to a small brain area called the median eminence (bottom of Figure 3) which connects the **pituitary gland** to the brain. This median eminence has unusually leaky blood vessels, so that insulin can escape from them and diffuse into the brain. This process can actually be seen, as a matter of fact. The bottom of Figure

Left: Figure 3. A mouse brain, shown in cross section. Top: Low-magnification view. The cerebral cortex covers the top of the brain, the hippocampus is just below the cortex (dense, dark-staining layers of neurons), and the hypothalamus is at the bottom of the brain. Middle: Higher-magnification view of the hypothalamus, showing the arcuate nucleus (1), the ventromedial nucleus (2), and the median eminence (arrow). Bottom: High-magnification view of the median eminence alone, showing radioactive molecules of insulin (points of light) diffusing upward into the hypothalamus out of leaky blood vessels in the median eminence.

3 shows the median eminence from a mouse that had been injected with trace amounts of insulin that had been made radioactive. Because of the radioactivity, each molecule of insulin can be detected and visualized and can be seen as a bright point of light passing from the median eminence and up into the hypothalamus. If these molecules of insulin are not there to dampen the activity of hypothalamic neurons, a mouse will start to eat excessive amounts of food.

INSULIN AND OBESITY

There is no danger that a diabetic mouse will become obese, no matter how much it eats, because fat cells can't manufacture fats out of glucose in the absence of insulin. An untreated diabetic mouse will naturally just get thinner and thinner, no matter how much it eats. What happens, however, if feeding-stimulating nerve cells in the hypothalamus become overactive *in spite of* the presence of insulin in a nondiabetic animal?

The consequences of this are illustrated in Figure 4, which shows two rats from the same litter belonging to the so-called "Zucker fatty" genetic strain of rat. One of these rats has inherited a gene that somehow causes hypothalamic neurons to become overactive, in spite of the presence of insulin in the blood which should normally inhibit them. This rat eats 50 percent more than normal, and as a consequence has become enormously obese. Also, this unfortunate animal would still get fat even if it went on a diet and ate only as much or less than its brother or sister next to it who has not inherited the gene for obesity and thus remains slim. Cutting down the food intake of the fat rat would only partially reduce its obesity. The reason for this depends on the fact that muscle and fat respond to insulin in different ways.

One other well-known feature of Zucker rats is that they tend to have higher than normal levels of insulin in

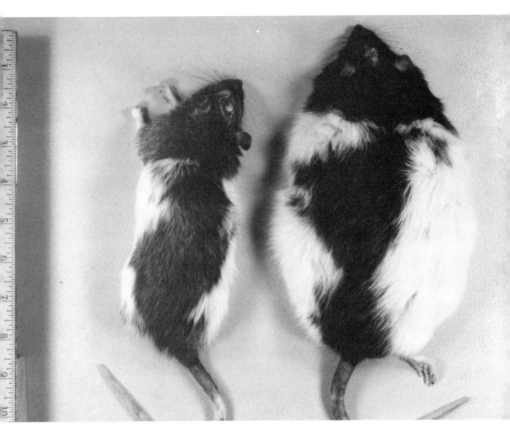

Figure 4. Two rats of the Zucker strain. The rat on the right has inherited a gene that causes obesity.

the blood. Recent work in the lab of a Swiss endocrinologist, Bernard Jeanrenaud, has shown that muscle and fat react to such an elevation in blood insulin in surprisingly different ways. Muscle cells adapt to elevated insulin by keeping their uptake (absorption) of glucose relatively constant or even below normal. Fat cells, in contrast, *increase* their glucose uptake four- or fivefold! That means that when a Zucker rat eats a cookie, the sugar in the cookie is five times more likely to be stored in fat than it would in a normal rat. Thus, both the overeating and the insulin-stimulated glucose metabolism in Zucker rats conspire to keep the rat fat. The actual gene or genes that cause these things to happen have still not been precisely identified.

OBESITY IN HUMAN BEINGS

We all know that some of us tend to gain weight no matter how much or how little we eat, whereas others stay slim in spite of "eating like a horse." Why is this? Do obese people have the same problems as the Zucker fatty rat?

The answer is yes and no.

One rather rare genetic disorder in humans does somewhat resemble the situation seen in Zucker rats. This disorder, called the Prader-Willi syndrome, is caused by an abnormal gene located somewhere on the tip of chromosome number 15 (see the beginning of Chapter Two for a brief discussion of chromosomes). Geneticists are rapidly learning more about this region of chromosome 15 and in the near future may precisely identify the gene affected in this syndrome. Features of this disorder become apparent in early childhood when a toddler starts to show signs of an unusually high level of hunger. Affected children will eat entire jars of mayonnaise or jam without stopping. To keep their weight within reasonable bounds, parents must face the distressing task of closely regulating the diet of children who are too young to understand the need for such restrictions. Like Zucker rats, Prader-Willi patients have elevated insulin levels and symptoms of hypothalamic dysfunction.

As for the rest of us, there is little reason to suspect gross abnormalities in hypothalamic function. For one thing, it is very difficult to show that most obese people eat appreciably more calories than lean people, in spite

20

of many studies trying to explore this possible reason for obesity. In a way, this should not be surprising.

In order to avoid getting fat, we all mainly need to eat only just as many calories as we burn to keep moving and to maintain bodily functions. If we eat just 5 percent more calories each day than we actually need, it is only a matter of time before such calories appear on our waistlines as fat. So, even small increases in food intake or, alternatively, slightly greater efficiency in burning the calories we eat, can eventually lead to the noticeable differences in the amount of fat between one person and another that can be seen in any gathering of people. The fact is, the basic causes of obesity are still not well understood.

One interesting study recently performed by Albert Stunkard at the University of Pennsylvania gives some insight into the influence of genetic inheritance upon obesity. Stunkard examined the medical records of some 4,000 servicemen. Half of these men were pairs of identical twins; the other half were pairs of fraternal twins raised in the same conditions. (Unlike identical twins, fraternal twins are not genetically identical). It turned out that if one identical twin became obese over time, his brother would also almost always get fat. On the other hand, fraternal twin brothers would get fat or remain thin over time, but the body weights of fraternal brothers would only occasionally change in the same way. This suggests that genetic inheritance, rather than environment or mode of upbringing, has the predominant effect in determining whether or not a person will get fat.

It has been known for years, from work on animals, that the hypothalamus regulates food intake and insulin levels so that the amount of fat on a given animal tends to remain pretty much the same over time. Hypothalamic nerve cells appear to do this by sending messages directly down nerve cell processes that end upon the surfaces of islet cells and also upon fat cells, regulating their activity.

Perhaps genetic mechanisms have directed the hypothalamus of each of us to maintain our own level of obesity, which is no more easy to change than our height, eye color, or body temperature.

CAUSES OF HUMAN DIABETES

Although the discovery of insulin was a major step in the treatment of diabetes, it is far from the final answer. Diabetics are no longer in immediate danger of dying, but insulin injections don't control levels of blood glucose as accurately or continuously as "home-grown" insulin from the islets. Fluctuations in blood glucose are thought to lead to abnormalities in blood vessels, causing tiny breaks and weaknesses in vessels in organs such as the retina of the eyes, the heart, and in body areas far from the heart like the feet. For these reasons, diabetes is considered one of the leading causes of heart disease and blindness in the United States. Also, many diabetics develop problems with their feet because of impaired circulation. These problems may become so bad that gangrene may set in and toes may have to be amputated; diabetes accounts for 40,000 amputations carried out each year. Obviously, diabetes should be prevented rather than simply treated with insulin. This cannot be accomplished until the causes of diabetes are understood.

JUVENILE-ONSET (TYPE-I) DIABETES

As it turns out, diabetes mellitus in humans is not just one simple disease, but comes in two rather different forms. About 10 percent of diabetics develop the disease in childhood and suffer from very low insulin production by islet cells. In this form of diabetes, known as juvenile-onset (or type-I) diabetes, islet cells fail to work because they are actually under attack by lymphocytes. Lymphocytes are cells of the immune system that normally act to fight disease by fighting bacteria. In type-I diabetes, these cells have turned against the islets of the body. Why?

The explanation is not yet known precisely. The substance in islet cells that is provoking the attack was identified in 1990. This substance is an islet cell protein called glutamic acid decarboxylase. The very presence of this material in islet cells itself was a surprise: the only other cells in the body that make it are *nerve cells* in the brain. Islet cells appear to make it as a "leftover" substance that they first began making early in development in the embryo: early in life, both nerve cells and islet cells appear to develop from a common "parent" cell. This is actually not as surprising as you might think. The function of both nerve cells and of hormone-producing cells is to communicate information. Nerve cells do this by secreting chemicals (transmitters) from long cell processes, and endocrine cells do this by secreting chemicals into the blood.

Why the immune system attacks this islet substance in the first place, leading to islet cell death, is still a mystery. But now, at least, the stage has been set for a basic understanding of type-I diabetes.

ADULT-ONSET (TYPE-II) DIABETES

About 90 percent of diabetics tend to develop their symptoms later in life, and while they, too, experience insufficient actions of insulin, their problems are not caused by a simple *lack* of insulin. Their islet cells show irregularities in timing of insulin release, along with a diminished *sensitivity* to insulin of muscle and fat cells that prevents insulin from working normally. The reasons why this insensitivity to insulin develops are not yet known. Another peculiarity of type-II diabetics is that their islet cells produce abnormally large amounts of a substance called amylin (EY-mi-lin) that accumulates outside of the cells and forms dense deposits. Such deposits were first recognized as long ago as 1905. Even now, however, the precise role of this amylin in the development of diabetes is still hotly debated: is it a cause, or only a result, of type-II diabetes mellitus? Further study should tell.

FINAL THOUGHTS ABOUT THE ISLETS OF LANGERHANS

All of the above have focused just on the insulin-producing cells of the islets, called beta (BAY-ta) cells. While they make up about 85 percent of all islet cells, they are not the only ones present. Other cells in the islets make a variety of less well-studied hormones. One particularly prominent one is **glucagon** (GLOOK-a-gon), which causes blood glucose levels to go *up* by reducing cell uptake of sugar. The cells that make glucagon, called alpha cells, rarely function incorrectly and only occasionally may cause disease. They are located around the outermost edges of each circular cluster of islet cells. Researcher L. Orci in Switzerland has demonstrated a fascinating property of islet cells: they all seem to "know" precisely where they "belong" in relation to one another. If islets are isolated, grown in a dish, and gently shaken apart, the separated cells will migrate together again and rearrange themselves so that the alpha cells once more occupy only the outer surface of each islet. Future study of these fascinating endocrine organs will doubtless show how this is accomplished, and how islet cells are related to diabetes in humans.

T W O
SEX HORMONES

Sex hormones are of obvious interest to all of us because they are partly responsible for "what makes the world go round": the sex differences in physical appearance and behavior that are part of why men and women are attracted to each other. Beyond this function in humans, sex hormones are tightly connected to a much more ancient function that arose early in evolution: the sexual mode of reproduction.

FEMALE SEX HORMONES: ESTROGEN AND PROGESTERONE

Sex hormones in women are mainly produced by the ovaries, organs that are entirely devoted to a most important task: the production of new human beings. To accomplish this, ovaries must act both as endocrine organs and as nurturing organs that shelter and nourish developing egg cells.

In Figure 5, a highly magnified view of an ovary can be seen. The most striking feature in this picture is the egg cell, or **oocyte** (OH-oh-site), one of the largest cells produced by the human body. The ovary of a young woman contains some 500,000 oocytes, each surrounded, nourished, and protected by cells called follicle cells. Each oocyte contains a large cell nucleus and an enormous volume of **cytoplasm**.

When the oocyte is later fertilized, genetic material in the sperm and egg cells will mix together and form a new cell nucleus that will divide many times and ultimately form a developing baby. Because a baby inherits genetic material (**genes**) from both the mother (oocyte) and father (sperm cell), each baby represents a unique combination of some of the features of each parent. This is made possible by combining twenty-three **chromosomes** (long molecules of **DNA**, or deoxyribonucleic acid) from the egg and sperm cells into twenty-three *pairs* of chromosomes that are found in each cell nucleus in a baby. Each of these twenty-three pairs of chromosomes is made up of one chromosome from the father and one from the mother. The information that determines how a baby will be formed is "written" in a sort of "code" on thousands of genes in each chromosome. The genes thus determine the anatomical and functional features of each of us.

All of this happens much later, after the oocyte has been released from the ovary in the process called **ovulation** (ov-yu-LAY-shun). Before this can happen, the oocyte must develop in a protective cocoon of follicle cells that surround it. It is these follicle cells that make the ovarian sex hormones.

The fact that the ovaries make hormones is something that became known relatively recently. The presence of egg cells in ovaries was discovered long ago, in 1672, by the Dutch anatomist Regner de Graaf. It was not until 1924, however, that the presence of the first known ovar-

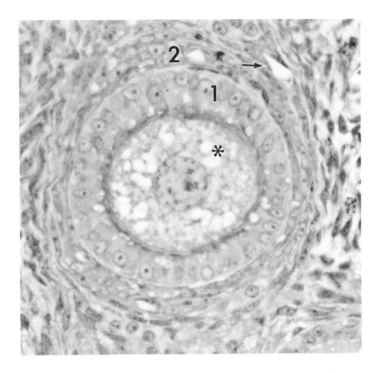

Figure 5. Cells in an ovary. The cytoplasm of an egg cell (*), nurturing granulosa cells (1), hormone-producing theca cells (2), and a small blood vessel (arrow) can be seen.

ian hormone was discovered. This breakthrough was accomplished by Edgar Allen and Edward Doisy, working at Washington University in St. Louis. They were able to isolate a substance from pig ovaries that had the properties of a hormone. This substance, which they called "oestrin," is nowadays known as **estrogen** (ES-tro-jen) and is responsible for the maintenance of uterine growth and function and for many of the sex differences in anatomy and physiology found in humans.

Two types of follicle cells can be seen in Figure 5. The type located closest to the oocyte and having tall, boxlike shapes are called **granulosa** (gran-yu-LO-sa) **follicle cells**. These cells mainly act to provide nourishment and guide the development of the oocyte. The second type are called **theca** (THEE-ka) **follicle cells**, and are the ones that manufacture estrogen. This layer of cells contains abundant numbers of blood vessels that carry the estrogen to all parts of the body.

EFFECTS OF ESTROGEN UPON THE BODY

Estrogen affects the function and appearance of the body in numerous and powerful ways. It enhances the deposition of fat beneath the skin. This is true all over the body, and accounts for the fact that women tend to have more body fat than men. But estrogen particularly stimulates accumulation of fat in the areas of the breasts and thighs. Estrogen makes a woman's skin smoother and thinner than a man's. One sex difference in anatomy that is even more prominent, even if it does not first come to mind, is the fact that women are shorter than men, due to the ability of estrogen to counteract the lengthening of limb bones that growth hormone would otherwise provoke. At the same time, however, estrogen has an opposite effect upon the bones of the pelvis, causing them to become wider than those of men.

Thus, in one individual, estrogen promotes a dramatic accumulation of fat in some cells but little in others, causes increased growth in some bones but decreased growth in others, and decreases multiplication of skin cells but increases multiplication of other cells, such as the cells forming the lining of the uterus! How can one hormone cause all these very different effects that almost magically sculpt the body and cause the changes that turn a girl into a woman? An even broader question relates to differences between individuals. Estrogen levels in the blood all tend to fall within a fairly narrow range for most women, suggesting that estrogen should have comparable effects in everyone. Yet, we all know that both men and women grow up to acquire great differences in height, shape, weight, etc. How can this be?

The only answer that can be given at this point is that individual cells, and individual people, have inherited genes that alter the ability to respond to estrogen. While great progress has been made in understanding how estrogen affects cells, we still have little knowledge of the mechanisms underlying this variability in the response to sex hormones. Even if we do not understand them, we can at least be grateful for their ability to permit the pleasing variability in the forms and features of the people around us.

REGULATION OF ESTROGEN AND PROGESTERONE SECRETION

Production of estrogen by theca cells is mainly controlled by two hormones secreted from the pituitary gland (see below) called **luteinizing** (LOO-tee-in-ai-zing) **hormone** (LH) and **follicle-stimulating hormone** (FSH). Most of the time, LH and FSH are secreted in rather constant amounts, and cause the production of a stable level of estrogen in the bloodstream. One additional effect of these basal levels of FSH is a gradual growth and enlargement of one or more follicles in the ovaries. About once a month, however, the brain stimulates the pituitary gland to secrete an enormous burst of LH called the LH surge. A rapid rise in FSH levels also occurs at this time. This massive outpouring of LH has a transforming effect upon the follicle cells. First, they become more loosely connected to each other, weakening the entire ovarian follicle and allowing the oocyte to burst through the surface of the ovary into the abdominal cavity. This event is called ovulation.

Next, the oocyte is transported down tubular organs called the uterine tubes, where it may or may not be fertilized by a sperm cell, and finally is carried into the interior of the uterus.

In the meantime, the follicle cells remaining in the ovary have not been idle but have produced a second response to the LH surge. Follicle cells multiply like mad and group together to form a large organ, the **corpus luteum** (KOR-pus LOO-te-um). This new organ growing within the ovary was first described in 1673 in cow ovaries by the Italian anatomist Marcello Malpighi, who called it the "yellow body" in Latin because in cows, unlike in women, it contains a distinctly yellow substance. Due to the work of George Corner in 1928, we now know that the transformed follicle cells of the corpus luteum produce another sex hormone, **progesterone** (pro-JES-ter-own).

Progesterone has a variety of its own effects, many of which cancel or modify the actions of estrogen and which prepare the uterus for taking care of a growing baby. Progesterone, for example, reduces muscular contractions of the uterus and stimulates uterine glands to secrete substances that may nourish or affect the development of a baby. The corpus luteum secretes progesterone for about thirteen days. If an embryo starts developing, it produces its own form of LH (detectable in the urine of a pregnant woman in so-called pregnancy tests) that keeps the corpus luteum functioning. If pregnancy does not begin, the corpus luteum, for reasons which are still largely mysterious, spontaneously degenerates, or "self-destructs."

When the corpus luteum degenerates, progesterone is no longer made. This has a disastrous effect upon the lining of the uterus. Cells in this lining stop secreting things, their blood supply becomes inadequate, and they die. In most mammalian species, these are about the worst effects of a fall in progesterone. In humans and a few species of monkeys, however, this cell damage is accompanied by a massive rupture and death of uterine blood vessels, leading to the extensive bleeding called **menstruation** (men-stroo-A-shun). Surprisingly, the reasons why the human uterus, and not the organs of other species, react in this way, are not clearly understood: why should uterine bleeding be important and necessary in humans but not in other animals? More study of the human uterus will be necessary to answer this question. After four to five days of bleeding, the damage is repaired and this whole sequence of events, called the ovarian cycle, begins again.

PUBERTY AND MENOPAUSE

The function of the ovaries changes dramatically with age; yet, the reasons for these changes are still not well understood. The beginnings of estrogen secretion, LH secretion, ovulation, and menstruation in girls typically starts around the age of twelve, but can begin as late as age fifteen. Why do these changes, called **puberty** (PYOO-ber-ty), begin?

The causes of puberty are difficult to study, for several reasons. Study of experimental animals such as rats has been helpful, but reproduction in these animals is not precisely like that in humans, so it is difficult to apply these findings to humans. Studies of puberty in rhesus monkeys, which are more like humans, have produced a variety of interesting results. Work done by Dr. Tony Plant at the University of Pittsburgh has shown that changes in the activity of nerve cells in the hypothalamus appear to initiate puberty by increasing the secretion of LH from the pituitary gland. What causes this maturation of hypothalamic nerve cells is unclear. Curiously, this process appears sensitive to the nutritional state of a monkey: if a monkey is given a restricted diet, puberty will be delayed.

These data in monkeys show a certain "logic" in the endocrine system: if not enough food is available to fatten up a monkey, then it certainly doesn't "make sense" to initiate puberty and the risks of a pregnancy. These monkey data are also consistent with the known delay of puberty that has been found in human populations exposed to periods of famine. However, how does the hypothalamus "know" that the body is too undernourished for reproduction? Perhaps insulin, affecting cell function in the hypothalamus, regulates the hypothalamic control of puberty as well as food intake.

At the other end of life, at ages forty-five to fifty, the ovarian cycles of a woman become more irregular and finally cease, a process known as **menopause**. Once again, the reasons for menopause are not at all well understood. Work in rats suggests that the ovaries are not at fault: if ovaries from older rats are transplanted into younger rats, they resume a normal function. Many people suspect that changes in the hypothalamus are again to blame, but what exactly happens is still unclear. Dr. Hyman Schipper, at a research institute in Montreal, has suggested one unorthodox explanation. He and coworkers have found that estrogen causes the production of a damaging chemical, called peroxidase, in the hypothalamus. With each cycle and each rise in blood levels of estrogen, more and more hypothalamic peroxidase is produced, leading to increasing damage to nerve cells. Finally, after about 400 cycles, or the average reproductive span of a woman's life, so much damage has accumulated in the hypothalamus that the proper control of the ovarian cycle ceases. Whether Schipper's hypothesis will prove to be correct remains to be seen.

Regardless of the cause of menopause, the loss of ovarian hormones in older women has a disruptive, and even perhaps unhealthy, influence upon the remainder of life. Physicians have increasingly supported the administration of small doses of estrogen to replace the missing ovarian estrogen in older women, and have found that this combats the loss of minerals in bones with age and reduces the risk of heart disease. Thus, the use of sex hormones can improve both the quality and quantity of life in older women.

EFFECTS OF ESTROGEN UPON THE BRAIN

Estrogen and progesterone, like insulin, also affect brain function as well as the function of the rest of the body. But the chemical structure of estrogen is different from that of insulin. Therefore, unlike insulin, estrogen can readily pass through the blood-brain barrier and thus can freely enter the brain. Only certain nerve cells, however, can remove estrogen from the blood, accumulate it within cell nuclei, and respond to it. Once again, the places in the brain where estrogen acts can be identified by making the estrogen radioactive and seeing where in the brain the radioactive molecules accumulate.

One area where estrogen acts is in the ventromedial nucleus of the hypothalamus (Figure 3). At this site, estrogen activates neurons that connect to the medulla and spinal cord and regulate sexual arousal and movement of back and pelvic muscles. Infusion of estrogen into this site stimulates female reproductive behavior in monkeys and rodents.

One additional effect of estrogen in this brain area is a reduction of food intake and appetite by about 20 percent. Presumably, this action of estrogen, and the ability of progesterone to reverse it, is related to the changes in appetite that can appear during pregnancy or during different phases of the ovarian cycle in women. There is some evidence that this ability of estrogen to affect appetite may contribute to the features of the self-starving disorder anorexia nervosa. In this disorder, patients proclaim that they feel too fat in spite of evidence to the contrary and may starve themselves down to 65 to 75 pounds. Anorexia primarily occurs in girls around the time of puberty and is perhaps related to a sudden rise in blood estrogen levels. This speculation is supported by the fact that occasionally girls treated with estrogen for a disorder called Turner's syndrome suddenly develop symptoms of anorexia. And these symptoms sometimes go away after estrogen therapy is stopped.

Yet another action of estrogen and progesterone upon the brain is the ability to affect body temperature by influencing nerve cells in other regions of the hypothalamus. A woman can take advantage of this effect to monitor when in the ovarian cycle ovulation occurs: the rise in progesterone that takes place soon after ovulation causes a rise in body temperature of about 2 degrees Fahrenheit that can be detected if body temperature is carefully measured each morning.

BIRTH CONTROL PILLS

The 1960s saw increased use of natural or synthetic forms of sex hormones to control fertility. Most of these drugs depend on estrogen's ability to suppress the secretion of LH. Because of this, the LH surge and the ovulation that it causes do not occur, and so no oocyte is available for fertilization. Since continuous stimulation of the uterus by either estrogen or progesterone is not desirable and can lead to irregular bleeding, many contraceptive preparations include "blank" pills that permit a regular process of menstruation once a month, in spite of the lack of an ovulation.

All of the above information serves to illustrate the many ways in which the ovaries are dedicated to the final goal of reproduction. Not only do the ovaries provide a nurturing environment for the oocytes, but they make hormones that provide the female body with sexual cues to attract a mate, prepare the body for pregnancy, and stimulate the brain to alter both sexual and feeding behavior in ways appropriate to prepare for reproduction.

MALE SEX HORMONES—TESTOSTERONE

Like the ovaries, the testes of men have two functions to perform: they must provide an environment for the development of sperm cells, and they must manufacture hormones. Sperm cells, like egg cells, are enclosed in a special cellular environment, this time in long, tortuous tubules called **seminiferous** (sem-in-IFF-er-os) **tubules**. Cross sections through these tubules can be seen in Figure 6. The hormone-producing cells are located in the spaces between these tubules, and are called **Leydig** (LIE-dig) **cells** after the German anatomist Franz Leydig, who first described them in 1850.

Studies of the endocrine function of the testis began in a rather unusual way in 1889 with the claim by the French physiologist Charles Brown-Sequard that extracts made from crushed dog testis had a rejuvenating effect upon him and other older men. This seemingly bizarre proposal was initially met with disbelief and derision, but succeeding studies proved the existence of a hormone from the testis. The existence of this hormone had been suspected from antiquity, since castration had long been known to make both animal and human males more feminine. Subsequent studies have shown that testosterone affects the body in many ways.

EFFECTS OF TESTOSTERONE UPON THE BODY

Most bodily effects of testosterone are the well-known changes that occur during puberty in boys. Testosterone increases the size of the testes, penis, and other, smaller glands within the abdomen such as the prostate that belong to the male reproductive system. Testosterone thickens the skin and causes beard growth. And at the same time, it can *decrease* hair growth on the head of some men so that they eventually can become bald! Once again, here is another example of how a sex hormone can have completely contradictory effects at two places in the

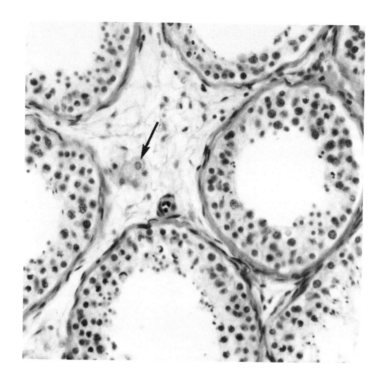

Figure 6. Cells in the testis. Circular cross sections of seminiferous tubules, where sperm cells mature, make up most of this view. One hormone-producing Leydig cell (arrow) can also be seen.

body that are separated from each other by only inches. And, once again, how do we explain how testosterone can reduce hair growth in some places of the body but not in others, and have this effect in some men but not in others? Our only (rather lame) explanation puts the blame on some unknown genes that some cells and people, but not others, have inherited.

One other effect that testosterone and similar hormones called **androgens** (AN-dro-jens) have is to somewhat increase muscular strength. In turn the bones are strengthened due to the increase in muscular tension upon them. This effect has led athletes to take huge doses of androgens to improve their performance. It is doubtful that the possible benefits of this practice outweigh the dangers. Careful tests of effects of androgens suggest that they really increase muscular strength by only a few percent. Some of the supposed benefits of androgens come from the so-called *placebo* (pla-SEE-bo) **effect**: athletes given ineffective placebo pills, thinking they were taking androgens, also tended to improve their strength and performance, perhaps because they trained harder to capitalize on their supposed androgen advantage.

The potential harmful effects of androgens, however, are clear. Androgens, like estrogens, also have the ability to prevent the secretion of pituitary hormones like LH and follicle stimulating hormone (FSH). This ability is part of the normal endocrine process called **negative feedback**, in which the sex hormones "tell" the pituitary not to make more LH and FSH than is needed to produce normal levels of estrogen or testosterone. When huge amounts of androgens are introduced into the body, LH and FSH secretion is almost totally shut down. Since LH and FSH are needed by the seminiferous tubules to produce sperm, androgens have the potential to produce temporary sterility by blocking sperm production. Also, as we shall see (Chapter Six), sex hormones have an ability to increase the risk for certain kinds of cancer. Finally, when large amounts of testosterone are introduced into the body, some of it is transformed into estrogen, which can then cause breast enlargement in males.

EFFECTS OF TESTOSTERONE ON THE BRAIN

Like estrogen, testosterone can have transient effects on the function of several brain areas. One additional surprising effect of testosterone is that it can not only affect the function of the brain but also its development and anatomy.

In Figure 7, cross sections through the hypothalamus of a male and female rat are shown. The difference between them is obvious: a cluster of nerve cells (arrows) is much larger in males than in females. Work in the laboratory of Roger Gorski at the University of California, Los Angeles (UCLA), has shown that this sex difference in brain anatomy appears to be due to the presence of male sex hormones at a certain stage of brain development in male rats. Later work has shown a similar effect of testosterone at other brain areas: for example, the spinal nerve cells that control the muscles of the genital area are more numerous in male rats.

When baby rats grow up, testosterone seems to act upon this same general area to stimulate male sex behavior. Thus, during development, testosterone provides for the development of a large collection of nerve cells that will later be activated by testosterone during adulthood.

These findings in rats may apply to humans as well, since similar sex differences in human brains have also been recently discovered. Dr. Simon LeVay in California has also reported that this brain area is relatively underdeveloped in homosexual men, and has suggested that a smaller stimulation of brain development by testosterone may be one reason for the altered sexual preference of adult homosexual men. More work needs to be done to prove whether such a simple hypothesis is true for a phenomenon as complex as sexual preference.

The regulation of sex behavior is clearly one brain function affected by testosterone. Another type of behavior, aggression, also seems subject to the influence of testosterone. Exposure of animals to testosterone, both during development and during adulthood, increases levels of aggressive behavior. This effect of testosterone may be related to the fact that the vast majority of murders in the world are committed by men. It is very difficult to

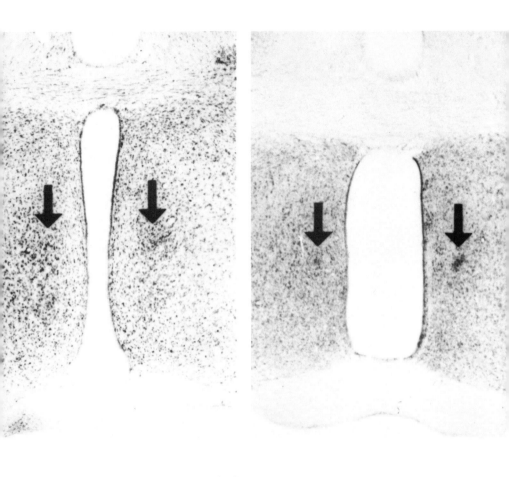

Figure 7. Hypothalamic cross sections from
a male (left) and female (right) rat. Arrows point
to groups of neurons that are larger in the male.

tell how much of this violent behavior comes from learning and upbringing and how much from hormones, but
hormones do appear to have some role in the sex differences in aggression.

Some behavioral scientists have speculated that aggressiveness in human males may be related to bodily effects of testosterone. Strength, for example, has a role in aggressive behavior. Even the presence of a beard may be indirectly related to aggression. Very few animals have large amounts of hair around the neck. One animal that does is the male lion; this hair helps minimize the damage done when two males fight, since the mane makes it difficult for bites into the neck to penetrate very far. Could a beard in human males have a similar primitive function? And if so, would it protect humans from other animals, or from other humans?

T H R E E

ADRENAL HORMONES

Another source of hormones in the body is the **adrenal glands**, which are small roughly pyramid-shaped organs located just above the kidneys. Because these glands are buried deep within the abdomen underneath all the gastrointestinal organs and are surrounded by abundant amounts of fat, they are difficult to locate.

The anatomy of the adrenals wasn't well described until the eighteenth century, but at that time their function couldn't even be guessed at. It wasn't until the pioneering work of an English physician, Thomas Addison, that it became clear that the adrenals are endocrine organs that can be involved in a number of diseases.

In 1855, Addison reported that a syndrome of extreme weakness, low blood pressure, weight loss, skin discoloration, and eventual death that he observed in a number of patients was accompanied by degeneration of the adrenals. He concluded that a new endocrine disorder was the explanation. This proposal led to a search for

41

adrenal hormones, which eventually yielded many more hormones than had actually been expected.

ADRENAL MEDULLA

As study of the adrenals progressed, it became clear that the hormonal activity present in each gland could be divided into two basic types, depending upon which region of the gland was extracted. Extracts of the *inner* portion of the gland, the medulla (muh-DUL-la), had rapid effects upon physiological functions such as the control of blood pressure. This effect was first discovered in 1893, when an English physician named George Oliver paid a visit to a physiologist, Edward Schaeffer, to show him an extract of adrenal medulla that he had made. Schaeffer at the time was in the middle of an experiment on the control of blood pressure in a dog and was irritated at the interruption. Oliver persevered, however, maintaining that after giving the extract to one of his patients, he came to the conclusion that the extract could affect blood pressure or heart rate. To mollify his friend, Schaeffer indulged him and let him administer the extract to the dog. Schaeffer then had to swallow his initial skepticism when the dog's blood pressure dramatically rose, indicating the presence of a previously unknown hormone! Many studies followed this initial observation, and a year later, in 1897, John Abel at Johns Hopkins was able to obtain pure crystals of this medullary hormone, which he named **epinephrine** (e-pi-NEF-rin). This name appears to come from a preference for Greek over Latin: *epi-nephros* is the Greek way of saying "above the kidney," as opposed to the Latin version *ad-renal* or *suprarenal*, which is more commonly used to describe these endocrine organs.

The top panel of Figure 8 shows the appearance of the cells in the adrenal medulla, which are clustered around large blood vessels into which they secrete their hormone. You may notice that some of these cells appear darker than others. This is because, after treatment with certain chemicals, a slightly modified form of epinephrine can be seen in about half of these cells. This form, called norepinephrine, attracts some cell stains more intensely and thus causes the cytoplasm of norepinephrine-containing cells to stain more darkly. Norepinephrine and epinephrine both increase heart rate and blood pressure, reduce stomach contractions, and affect other organs when secreted into the bloodstream from the adrenal medulla. The medulla is generally stimulated to secrete upon commands from the nervous system, carried by nerves that end on medullary cells.

More recently, a new hormone has been discovered in medullary cells that secrete epinephrine. This hormone, called enkephalin (en-KEF-a-lin), has the ability to block sensations of pain by binding or attaching to the cell membranes of nerve cells. The existence of these enkephalin-sensitive, painkilling sites on nerve cells, or enkephalin receptors, explains why poppy extracts containing opium or heroin are able to change our sensation of pain. The poppy plant appears to have evolved the ability to make opium as a defense against being eaten! After an animal eats poppies, the opium stimulates the enkephalin receptors in the animal's nervous system and makes the animal feel disoriented and strange. Such a poisoned animal is less likely to eat another poppy the next day. Drugs that mimic the effects of our own enkephalins have unfortunately provided society with the problems of drug addiction, in addition to the benefits of painkilling anesthetics.

ADRENAL CORTEX

Cells of the cortex, or outer portion, of the adrenal manufacture hormones with an entirely different structure and function. Hormones of the adrenal cortex are essential for

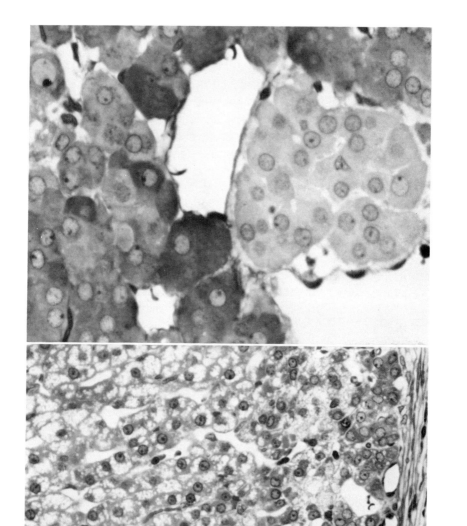

life; the absence of these hormones after surgical removal of the adrenals or in Addison's disease is the explanation for the shortened lifespan seen in these conditions. At least three types of adrenal cortical hormones are known: glucocorticoids, mineralocorticoids, and sex steroids.

An example of the first type is **cortisol**, which is termed a **glucocorticoid** (gloo-co-COR-ti-coid) because of its ability to raise levels of glucose in the blood. Glucocorticoids were first extracted from adrenals in 1930 by Frank Hartman, who was able to show their use as a hormone in cats whose adrenals had been removed. Later, in 1933, Edward Kendall was able to prepare pure crystals of a glucocorticoid and to eventually make large amounts of it. In 1948, Philip S. Hench, who worked with Kendall at the Mayo Clinic in Minnesota, obtained glucocorticoids from Kendall and administered them to patients with severe arthritis. This treatment proved amazingly effective, allowing severely crippled patients to suddenly resume walking without pain. At first, glucocorticoids were thought to be a "wonder drug" for arthritis; then, the euphoria subsided.

The reason for this renewed caution was an increasing understanding of the effects of glucocorticoids. The basis for these hormones' beneficial effects upon arthritis is their ability to prevent inflammation and tissue destruc-

Left: Figure 8. Top: High-magnification view of cells of the adrenal medulla that make norepinephrine (darker cells) and epinephrine (lighter cells). Bottom: Lower-magnification view of cells in the adrenal cortex. The darker cells at far right primarily make aldosterone, whereas the cells containing more lipid droplets primarily make cortisol.

tion by cells of the immune system. However, other, negative effects are also prominent: glucocorticoids cause the breakdown of tissue components such as **proteins** and their conversion into glucose, raising levels of glucose in the blood. This eventually weakens the structure of skin and muscle. These symptoms, in fact, occur naturally when the adrenal gland makes too many glucocorticoids, a syndrome first identified in 1912 by the American physician Harvey Cushing. For this reason, glucocorticoids cannot safely be given to people in large doses for long periods, and thus are only temporary "cures" for inflammatory diseases like arthritis.

An example of a second type of adrenal cortical hormone is **aldosterone** (al-DOS-ter-own), which is termed a **mineralocorticoid** (min-er-al-o-COR-ti-coid) because it alters the metabolism of the mineral sodium in our bodies. Aldosterone acts on the kidney to prevent the loss of sodium in the urine; without aldosterone, normal balances of sodium and water in the body are disrupted, blood pressure falls, and the circulatory system "collapses." Aldosterone is clearly one adrenal hormone that is necessary for life.

Finally, a third function of the adrenal cortex is to make small amounts of sex hormones like estrogen and testosterone. We are not certain why this additional source of sex hormones is necessary, and what role these adrenal sex hormones normally play in puberty and reproduction. Occasionally, the adrenals may make too many of these hormones in a disorder called the adreno-genital syndrome. This can result in early puberty or a masculinizing effect upon affected women.

Cells of the adrenal cortex are shown in the bottom panel of Figure 8. The outermost cells primarily make aldosterone. Cells located further into the cortex make glucocorticoids and often appear filled with small bubbles when viewed through the light microscope. In life, these "bubbles" are actually little droplets of oil, or lipid.

46

These adrenal cells need lots of lipid because the hormones they make—aldosterone, glucocorticoids, and sex hormones—are all **steroid hormones**, made by slightly changing the shape and atoms of a lipid molecule called cholesterol. Adrenal medullary hormones, in contrast, are formed by slightly modifying the atoms in a nonfatty substance, an **amino acid** called tyrosine. The chemical natures and modes of action of these and other hormones will be discussed further in Chapter Six.

THE ADRENAL GLANDS AND STRESS

After reviewing all these adrenal hormones, one logical question would be: what purpose do these compounds serve? Why would a single gland produce hormones that have so many apparently unrelated effects, like increasing heart rate and blood glucose and decreasing sensitivity to pain?

The answer can follow from imagining a stressful situation. Let's suppose you are taking a walk in the woods, and you spot a wolf far away. The wolf looks at you, you look at it, and your nervous system signals your adrenal medulla to release epinephrine. Your heart beats faster and supplies muscles (leg muscles and others) with more blood so they can start running away. After a while, you look over your shoulder and notice the wolf is following you! This time, your brain stimulates the pituitary gland to release a hormone called **adrenocorticotropic hormone** (*ACTH*). ACTH is carried to the adrenal cortex, causing it to release glucocorticoids that raise blood levels of glucose and thus provide your muscles with more fuel so that they can sustain their effort.

All is in vain, however, because the wolf gets close enough to momentarily nip you on the leg! Normally, you might bend down, rub your ankle, and say "Gee, that smarts!" Now, however, is not the time for this, so released enkephalins from the adrenal medulla prevent you from noticing the pain and keep you running onward to safety. Also, your leg won't swell up from inflammation, because glucocorticoids prevent this. Adrenal androgens could possibly help your morale and keep up your fighting spirit by enhancing aggressiveness. All these actions of adrenal hormones would have a bad effect on the body if continued indefinitely. In an emergency, though, they allow you to ignore short-term needs and consequences so that you can escape to safety.

EFFECTS OF ADRENAL CORTICAL HORMONES ON THE BRAIN

Brain effects of adrenal corticoids are less well studied than those of other hormones, but some influences upon behavior are known. One example is that corticoids seem to increase the ability of rats to learn and remember things. Since these hormones are often secreted in response to stress or danger, the value of an increased memory in these circumstances is obvious. One recent and astonishing finding, reported by R. S. Sloviter and co-workers at Columbia, was that removal of the adrenals in rats causes 70 percent of the nerve cells in a certain portion of the hippocampus to die and permanently disappear. The hippocampus (see top of Figure 3 on page 16), a brain structure known to participate in processes of learning and memory, may be damaged in people with memory disorders and Alzheimer's disease. Thus, more study of effects of adrenal hormones upon this structure will probably follow.

F O U R

THYROID AND PARATHYROID HORMONES

Another endocrine organ of great interest is the **thyroid gland**, which is located in the neck just below the shield-shaped cartilages that enclose the larynx (*thyroid* is Greek for "shield"). The thyroid is a soft gland with two lobes that is wrapped around the trachea (windpipe) and that appears reddish pink in the fresh condition, due to the many blood vessels that pass through it. The existence and anatomy of this gland has been well known since it was first described in 1656 by the English physician Thomas Wharton, who gave it its name. (Wharton's *Adenographia* gave the first thorough account of the glands of the human body.) Its function, however, was uncertain; Wharton suggested that it might lubricate the larynx and sweeten the voice!

Even in Wharton's time, however, there was a lot of evidence that the thyroid was involved in far more serious and important functions than this. An abnormally enlarged thyroid gland, in fact, was known to be a symptom of serious disease by both Roman and ancient Chinese physicians. Unlike other endocrine organs such as the pancreas and adrenals, the importance of the thyroid was established in antiquity. A basic problem in progressing beyond this was the fact that an enlarged thyroid, or **goiter** (GOY-ter), was present in *two* diseases that were absolutely unlike! Why would two diseases with different symptoms—simple goiter and toxic goiter—both be associated with an enlarged thyroid?

A look at the two main thyroid diseases shows how perplexing this problem was. In the first type, simple goiter, the symptoms were an enlarged thyroid, short height, puffiness of the face, obesity, and a slow heartbeat and metabolic rate. If the disease began in a newborn infant, the child would grow up with severe mental retardation, a condition called "cretinism." In the second type, toxic goiter, the symptoms were an enlarged thyroid, extreme slenderness, rapid heart rate, accelerated metabolism, and a "pop-eyed" appearance resulting from an expansion of tissue behind the eyes that pushed the eyeballs forward in the orbital cavities (see Figure 9). How could an enlarged thyroid possibly cause *both* of these puzzling conditions?

THYROID HORMONE PRODUCTION

This puzzle can only now be understood, thanks to progress in understanding how the thyroid gland makes thyroid hormone, called **thyroxine** (thy-ROX-in). Cells of the thyroid are shown in Figure 10. These cells, called follicle cells, are attached to each other to form hollow spheres, called follicles, that contain fluid in their centers. Each cell makes some of the fluid, and secretes into the fluid a large molecule called **thyroglobulin**. Thyroglobulin is a protein, that is, a very long chain of dozens of simple molecules called amino acids. Small fragments of this long molecule at some times are removed from the thyroglobulin and secreted into nearby capillaries as thyroxine.

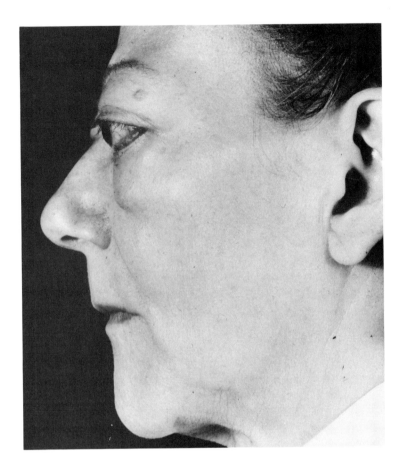

Figure 9. Patient with toxic goiter (also known as hyperthyroidism), a disease characterized by protruding eyeballs and weight loss

To make thyroxine, follicle cells modify some of the thyroglobulin and then break it into fragments. First, the follicle cells actively take up iodine atoms from the blood and attach them to certain amino acids (tyrosine amino acids) that are part of the chain that makes up thyroglobulin (Figure 11). Next, two of the iodinated ty-

51

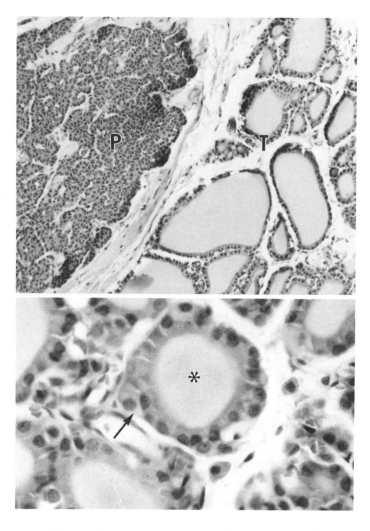

Figure 10. Top: Low-magnification view of
thyroid tissue (T) and part of the parathyroid gland
(P) that adheres to the back of the thyroid gland.
Bottom: Thyroid follicle cells, grouped
around fluid containing thyroglobulin (*).
A few lighter-staining parafollicular
cells (arrow) can also be seen.

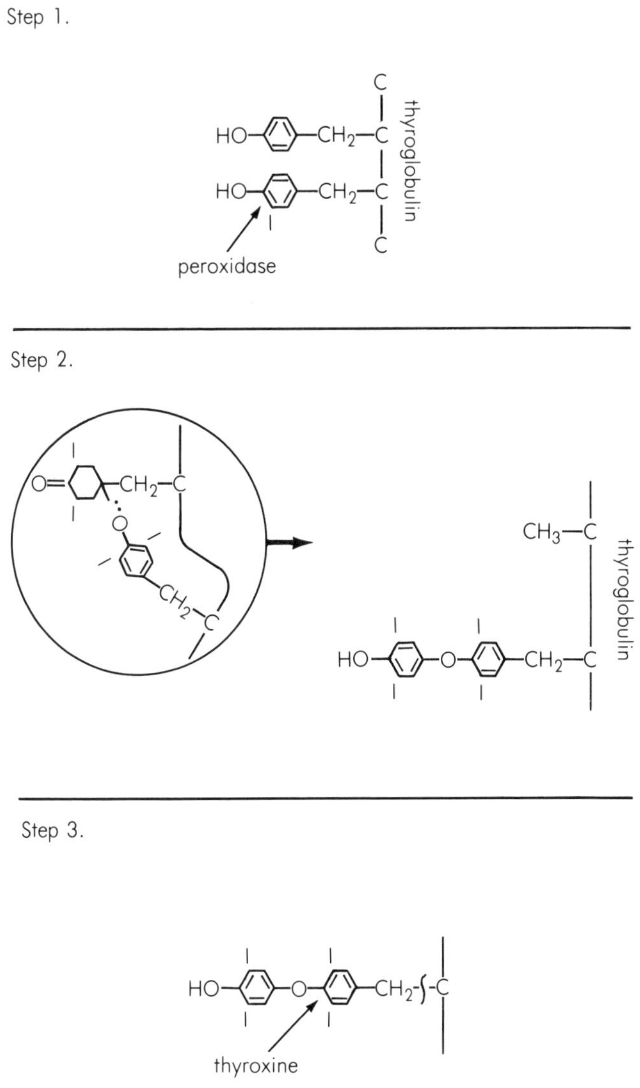

Figure 11. How the thyroid gland produces thyroxine (T4).

rosines are joined together, and then these joined, iodi-nated tyrosines are broken off from the thyroglobulin protein and are secreted into the bloodstream as a hor-mone. This hormone, containing four atoms of iodine, is called tetraiodothyronine, or for short, thyroxine.

Believe it or not, once this completed biochemical story was understood, the explanations for the two types of thyroid disease became obvious.

The cause of simple goiter is a deficiency of iodine in food and drinking water. When the thyroid lacks iodine, it can't manufacture thyroxine, so blood levels of thyroxine fall. It turns out that the hypothalamus appears to keep a close "watch" on thyroxine levels, so when they fall too low, the hypothalamus stimulates the pituitary gland to secrete a hormone called **thyroid-stimulating hor-mone (TSH)**, which is designed to stimulate the thyroid and make sure it's doing its job. This is just another example of the principle of negative feedback (see sec-tion on androgens in Chapter Two). In this example of negative feedback, a low level of thyroxine "tells" the brain and pituitary that the thyroid gland is not function-ing properly and, as a result, more TSH is produced. The thyroid responds to the TSH by trying to make more thyroxine. It gets bigger and bigger, but because there is no iodine all is in vain. The other symptoms of simple goiter result from thyroxine deficiency.

EFFECTS OF THYROXINE ON THE BODY AND BRAIN

Normal thyroxine, containing iodine, has a stimulatory effect on heartbeat and metabolic rate; a deficiency of it therefore explains the slow heartbeat, obesity, and puffi-ness seen in simple goiter. Also, thyroxine is necessary for normal brain development, so an absence of it in new-borns can cause mental retardation. Fortunately, babies are nowadays quickly examined at birth for thyroxine in the blood; if it is too low, administration of thyroxine during the first five months after birth can restore a normal IQ to over three fourths of affected infants.

This modern knowledge of simple goiter also explains some puzzling findings of eighteenth- and nineteenth-century medicine. From antiquity, it had been known that eating seaweed tended to cure symptoms of simple goiter, but it was not until the 1820s that the French physicians Bernard Courtois and Jean Coindet discovered that seaweed contained iodine and that iodine itself could be used to treat simple goiter. This use of iodine became so popular, in fact, that by 1859 Frederic Rilliet of Geneva published a paper warning about the toxic effects of giving too much iodine to people. The reason why iodine worked was not really clear until Edward Kendall (the same Kendall who later isolated adrenal hormones) made pure crystals of thyroxine on Christmas Day, 1914, and found that the hormone itself required iodine for biological activity. This would eventually lead to the ability to give thyroxine itself, instead of iodine, to some patients, although this step had to come much later, after improved methods of extracting or manufacturing thyroxine were worked out: by early methods, 3 tons of pigs' thyroids had to be processed to obtain only 30 *grams* of thyroxine!

What about the other type of goiter, toxic goiter? It turns out that this results from a thyroid that has become enlarged and overactive rather than underactive, producing too much thyroxine and stimulating overall metabolism too much. The reasons for this type of thyroid disease are entirely different: in toxic goiter, thyroid cells are attacked by cells of the immune system, rather like in type-I diabetes. Instead of being destroyed, however, thyroid cells are stimulated. Why?

Recent evidence suggests that the part of thyroid cells under attack are the sites on the cell membrane where TSH attaches. In toxic goiter, immune system cells make

55

chemicals called **antibodies** that themselves attach to these TSH-sensitive sites. The thyroid cells can't tell the difference between antibodies attaching to these sites and TSH attaching to the sites. They respond as if TSH were instructing them to make more thyroxine, and so become hyperactive. The reasons why the immune system would act upon the thyroid like this are not now known. An additional, and also unexplained, attack by immune cells upon the muscles that move the eyeball causes these muscles to become inflamed and enlarged, pushing the eyes forward in their sockets. Also, for unknown reasons, more women than men tend to develop this condition.

One way of curing toxic goiter takes advantage of the ability of the thyroid to accumulate large amounts of iodine by taking it up from the bloodstream. In 1939 it occurred to a Boston physician, Saul Hertz, that if slightly radioactive iodine were given to a patient, it would primarily accumulate in the thyroid, destroy the hyperactive cells, and leave other bodily organs unharmed. This approach has since been used with great success to treat thyroid overactivity without actual surgery.

CALCITONIN

In the last several decades it has become clear that the follicle cells of the thyroid are not the only ones that make a hormone. Other, pale-staining cells (Figure 10) also inhabit the thyroid gland; these cells neither contact, produce, nor alter thyroglobulin, and in fact have an entirely separate endocrine function. Because these cells lie beside the follicles, they were named **parafollicular cells** (*para* means "alongside" in Latin) by Jose Nonidez in New York in 1932. Nonidez also speculated that they may have an endocrine function, but his suggestion was virtually ignored for almost thirty years. Finally, in 1962, Douglas Copp and colleagues in Vancouver, Canada, reported the existence of a new hormone that they called

calcitonin (cal-si-TONE-in) because of its ability to lower blood concentrations of calcium. Two years later, Iain MacIntyre and Everson Pearse in England were able to conclusively show that this new hormone is produced by thyroid parafollicular cells.

As we shall see, it is extremely important that blood levels of calcium be precisely controlled, so that cells (such as nerve and muscle cells) function properly. Secretion of calcitonin is one way of controlling blood levels of calcium. How does calcitonin lower blood calcium, and where does this calcium disappear to?

The effects of calcitonin are related to the fact that we all carry with us a metabolic "calcium bank" that allows us to precisely regulate blood levels of calcium by making regular deposits or withdrawals of calcium. This "calcium bank" is the body's bone tissue. Calcium is withdrawn from bone by the action of specialized cells called **osteoclasts** (OSS-tee-o-clasts, "bone eaters").

Hormone-sensitive osteoclast cells are some of the most remarkable cells in the body. They arise when circulating blood cells called *monocytes* settle down upon the surface of a bone. For unknown reasons, these cells develop the ability to give up their individuality and then fuse together into one bizarre, giant cell that may contain as many as fifty cell nuclei! These cells then acquire the ability to destroy bone, which, as the body's "armor plate," is one of the most difficult substances to remove. Osteoclasts accomplish this by producing acid between themselves and the surface of the bone they are attached to. This acid environment dissolves the specialized form of calcium phosphate that is present in bone and thus removes the minerals that make bone hard. You can also perform your own experiment to duplicate this feat: if a chicken bone is placed in carbonated soda pop for several weeks, the weak acid in the soda will gradually remove the mineral in the bone, leaving only the protein, so that it becomes soft and flexible.

The last step in bone removal by osteoclasts is to also destroy the remaining bone proteins, which is achieved by specialized chemicals called enzymes that are secreted onto bone by the osteoclasts. The calcium released during this entire process is then free to enter the bloodstream. Calcitonin diminishes blood levels of calcium by restraining this action of osteoclasts. If calcium levels fall *too* low, however, parafollicular cells respond by not secreting calcitonin, thus allowing osteoclasts to go back to work again.

In the last ten years, this action of calcitonin upon osteoclasts has been found to be of aid in combatting a bone disease. In this disease, first described in 1876 by the English physician James Paget, osteoclasts are overactive and cause a progressive weakening of bones, particularly those in the spine, pelvis, and legs. Current evidence suggests that this is due to infection of osteoclasts with some sort of virus. This disorder is relatively common, affecting as many as 3 percent of all people over thirty-five, and produces variable degrees of bone deformities and pain due to bone compression. Administration of synthetic calcitonin, along with other drugs that diminish osteoclast activity, has been found to be highly effective in reducing the pain and bone weakness in Paget's disease.

PARATHYROID HORMONE

The long and puzzling quest for an understanding of the function of the thyroid gland was actually made even more difficult by the presence of other, tiny endocrine glands buried in the space between the thyroid gland and trachea. These glands (Figure 10), whose existence was not even suspected, proved responsible for some of the unexpected effects of thyroid gland removal. One such effect was first described by Moritz Schiff of Geneva in 1884. Schiff found that after thyroid removal, some animals would develop increasingly violent trembling of the muscles, called tetany, that could eventually even lead to death. More disturbingly, a percentage of patients who had undergone thyroid surgery to remove goiters would also develop these same deadly symptoms. What was their cause?

The search for the cause of tetany led to an enhanced scrutiny of thyroid anatomy. One example of these studies was that of the Swedish researcher Yvar Sandstrom, who first completely described the small, round parathyroid glands that could be found buried within the back surface of the thyroid in humans. It was not really surprising that these tiny glands had not been described in humans well before—in fact, they had only been discovered in 1852 by the British naturalist Richard Owen. Owen's main scientific interest was the anatomy of large animals, like the dinosaur fossils that he studied. In 1852 he also studied the anatomy of the Indian rhinoceros and came upon parathyroid glands that in this huge species, at least, were large enough to be noticeable.

These anatomical studies provided the first clues of the cause of tetany. The Italian researchers Giulio Vassale and Francisco Generali were then able to prove, in 1896, that accidental removal of the parathyroids during goiter surgery was the probable explanation for the symptoms of tetany seen in some patients. We now know that tetany results from the dramatic fall in blood levels of calcium that occurs when the parathyroids are removed. What, however, is the mechanism of this effect?

EFFECTS OF PARATHYROID HORMONE UPON CALCIUM METABOLISM

It was not until 1959 that the team of Rasmussen and Craig succeeded in extracting a hormone, **parathyroid hormone** (**PTH**), from cow parathyroids. We now know that PTH is a protein hormone composed of a chain of eighty-four amino acids that is secreted from parathyroid gland cells. These cells are gathered together in clusters that are richly supplied with blood vessels to carry the hormone away. PTH raises blood levels of calcium, once again, by acting upon osteoclasts. Instead of inhibiting osteoclast activity, like calcitonin, PTH *stimulates* their activity and increases the destruction of bone, releasing calcium into the blood.

Now that this effect of PTH is understood, it is easy to understand why parathyroid removal would lead to a drastic fall in blood concentrations of calcium. Why, however, would this lead to tetany? The explanation involves the spots, called neuromuscular junctions, at which nerves contact muscles to cause them to contract. When blood calcium falls too low, these neuromuscular junctions become too easily excited, leading to uncontrollable muscle twitches and convulsions. Tetany can thus be reversed by infusions of calcium into the bloodstream. This treatment is nowadays seldom necessary, since accidental removal of the parathyroids is always avoided during thyroid surgery.

An excess, rather than a deficiency, of PTH is another medical condition involving PTH that a physician is likely to encounter today. For example, tumors of the parathyroid glands can release large amounts of PTH and cause a general bone weakening. Also, in some types of cancer of bone marrow or of immune system cells—a cancer called multiple myeloma is a good example—the abnormal cells secrete some type of substance that mimics effects of PTH. As a result, patients with these types of cancer can experience painful fractures of spinal or leg bones. More study of PTH may perhaps lead to improved treatments for these conditions.

F I V E

PITUITARY HORMONES:

HORMONES THAT CONTROL OTHER HORMONES

One small, pea-sized gland that is locked away deep inside the human skull has the ability to produce ten separate hormones and has a commanding influence upon a dazzling variety of structures in the human body. This gland is the **pituitary gland**, and is illustrated in Figure 12. This drawing shows the appearance of the human brain and hypothalamus when cut in longitudinal section, that is, cut at a right angle to the plane of the cut illustrated in Figure 3 on page 16, so that the tip and handle of the knife would be located at the front and rear of the brain respectively. Figure 12 shows how the pituitary gland hangs suspended from the median eminence (see Figure 3 for a view of a cross section, rather than a longitudinal section, of the median eminence). The pituitary is positioned roughly midway between the anterior and posterior surfaces of the brain.

Much of the activity of the pituitary involves controlling the activity of other endocrine glands, in other words,

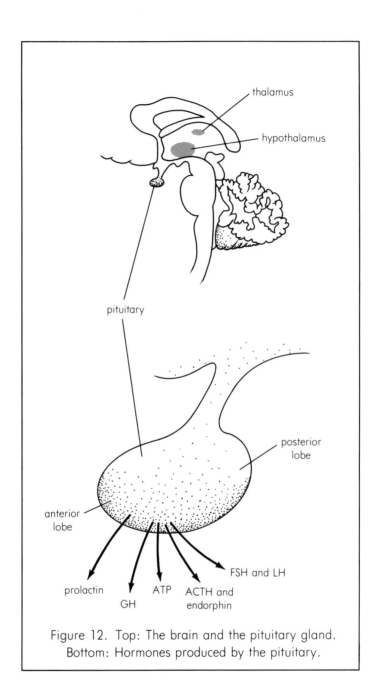

Figure 12. Top: The brain and the pituitary gland.
Bottom: Hormones produced by the pituitary.

producing hormones that control the production of other hormones. This controlling influence gives the pituitary an importance all out of proportion to its small size. This importance was not recognized for some time because the location of the pituitary made the study of its function almost impossible.

Oscar Minkowski's discovery in 1887 that a disorder of growth called *acromegaly* (aa-krow-MEG-a-lee) often occurred along with tumors of the pituitary was one early indication that the pituitary had an endocrine function. Minkowski must have been a very busy man, since he also discovered the importance of the pancreas in diabetes (see Chapter One). His observations suggested that the overactive pituitary was producing something that caused excessive growth of bones and soft tissues. It is now known that this was due to an overproduction of pituitary growth hormone (see below). Too much growth hormone in younger people can cause a general lengthening of bones and an excessive, "giant" height (Figure 13). In older people, bones have lost the ability to lengthen, so that growth hormone can only cause bone thickening, curvature of the spine, and enlarged brows, noses, and ears, which are features of acromegaly.

All this could only be guessed at in 1887. How could a role for the pituitary in acromegaly be proven? The obvious next step was to remove the pituitary in experimental animals and see if growth became slower. This, however, is more easily said than done!

The location of the pituitary, buried deep within the skull, makes it extremely hard to approach surgically. Harvey Cushing and other endocrinologists first tried to approach it from above by gently lifting and shoving aside the brain so that the pituitary could be removed in experimental animals. This approach, in spite of heroic efforts, was only rarely successful. In 1912 the Viennese researcher Bernard Aschner published a description of another approach, in which the pituitary gland could be

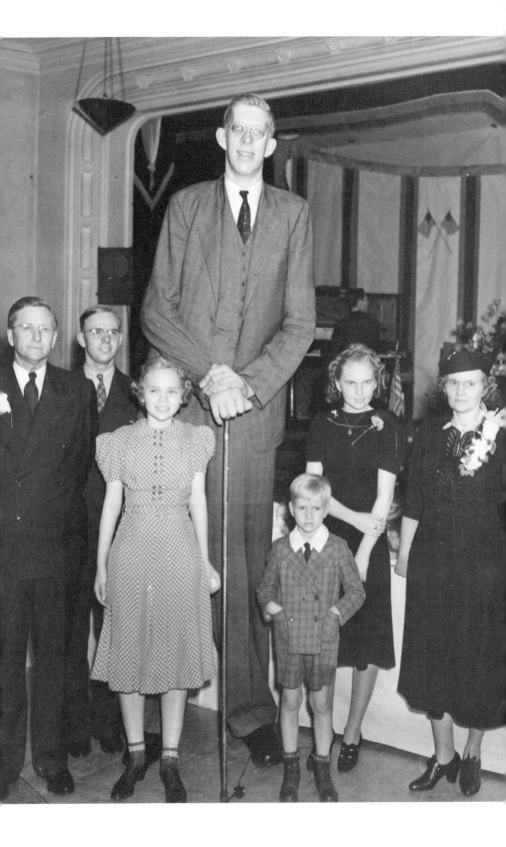

removed through a small hole cut through the bones forming the roof of the nasal cavity. This proved much more satisfactory, and Aschner was able to confirm an endocrine influence of the pituitary upon growth and also upon the size and activity of the adrenal and thyroid glands in dogs.

ANTERIOR PITUITARY HORMONES

Further examination of the pituitary showed that it is composed of a posterior lobe, produced by a down-growth from the brain during development, and an anterior lobe, produced by development of cells that originated in the mouth of the embryo. These two very different populations of cells grow toward each other during development and fuse to form the two portions of the adult gland. The endocrine activity of the gland can best be understood if the two lobes are considered separately.

Cells in the anterior lobe form irregular clusters that secrete hormones into nearby blood capillaries (see Figure 14). Some of the cells contain cytoplasmic granules that stain particularly dark with certain stains (arrows). These cells are called **basophils** (BAYZ-o-fils, Latin for "base-loving") because their granules stain well with certain dyes that are bases rather than acids. The granules that are stained represent little intracellular packages of hormones that are ready to be secreted into the environ-

Figure 13. Gigantism results from oversecretion of growth hormone. This 1939 photo shows Robert Wadlow, an 8-foot-8½-inch giant who lived in Illinois, celebrating his twenty-first birthday with members of his family.

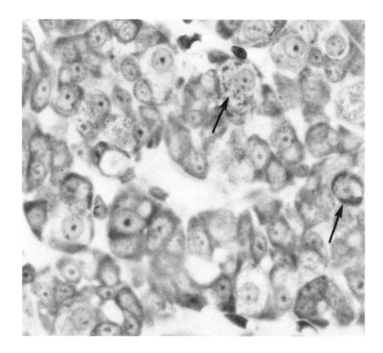

Figure 14. Anterior pituitary cells. Arrows indicate the dark-staining secretory granules of basophil cells, containing LH, FSH, TSH, or ACTH.

ment around the cell. Other cells in the anterior lobe also contain granules, but these granules don't stain as well, so that these cells, **acidophils** ("acid-loving"), may have a pale-staining cytoplasm.

Each basophil cell may produce and secrete one of six different hormones, which are all basically devoted to controlling other endocrine organs. Two of these hormones are LH and FSH, which, as we have said, control the activity of the ovaries and testes. Dr. James McKenzie has recently discovered that the cells that make LH and FSH may also contain atrial natriuretic peptide, a hormone that is also produced by the heart. What role this additional hormone plays in the control of reproduction by the pituitary represents yet another mystery in endocrinology. Another hormone produced by basophils is TSH, which, as we have seen, controls the activity of the thyroid gland.

One molecule produced by another type of basophil has a very complicated life story. This molecule, a protein with the improbably long name of **proopiomelanocortin** (pro-opee-o-mel-an-o-KOR-tin), is cut up into several fragments as soon as it is secreted. Each fragment then becomes a separate hormone. One fragment, called ACTH, stimulates the activity of the adrenal cortex. If adrenal cortical hormones become too low in the blood, these cells secrete more ACTH. Another fragment, secreted along with ACTH, is **melanocyte-stimulating hormone**, or MSH. MSH is very important in furry animals like weasels and rabbits, because by stimulating pigment-producing cells in the skin, it can aid in changing fur color from white back to brown again when winter changes into spring. In humans, MSH does not seem to have much influence, with one notable exception.

One remarkable symptom of adrenal failure, or Addison's disease, is that the color of the skin of Addison's patients tends to turn browner. The explanation for this is that the pituitary is secreting very high amounts of ACTH to "kick-start" the adrenals into activity again, and along with the ACTH, MSH is also secreted. MSH causes the skin to change color. This symptom of Addison's disease used to be of great importance to physicians in diagnosing the disorder, which often used to result from tubercular infections of the adrenal glands. Now that tubercular infections have become rarer, however, Addison's disease and its abnormal browning of the skin are rarely seen.

One final fragment produced by basophils was isolated by A. F. Bradbury and colleagues in 1975 and is called **endorphin** (en-DOR-fin). This protein hormone, like adrenal enkephalin, has the ability to bind to pain receptors in the nervous system. It too may be released from the pituitary gland in times of stress and may diminish our perception of pain. The ancient Chinese art of painkilling by acupuncture may, in fact, involve this hormone, since brain and blood levels of endorphin have been shown by English researchers to go up during acupuncture.

All these hormones, produced by anterior-lobe basophil cells, basically seem to be controllers of other endocrine glands. The hormones produced by acidophils, in contrast, were long regarded to have direct effects upon nonendocrine tissue.

GROWTH HORMONE

The first acidophil hormone to be studied in detail was growth hormone, or *somatotropin*. Growth-promoting activity of pituitary extracts was established during the 1920s, and by 1945 a purified growth-promoting hormone was obtained by C. H. Li in California. Studies of the purified hormone revealed one mechanism that accounted for the increased growth seen after injections of growth hormone (GH). This mechanism involves a specialized layer of cartilage, called the **epiphyseal** (eh-pi-fi-SEE-al) **plate**, that is present at the end of long bones like the femur in the leg. After an injection of GH, some of the cartilage cells in these plates start multiplying rapidly, so that they start to pile up on one another like stacks of coins (see Figure 15). Later, some of the cells swell up and eventually die, leaving behind thin plates of cartilage proteins that will become replaced by true bone. A result of this process is that the epiphyseal plate temporarily widens, pushing upon the end of the femur lying above it and causing the bone to lengthen a bit. Repetition of this process many times accounts for the growth that is seen after injections of GH.

By 1957 this process had become so well understood that two researchers, W. D. Salmon and W. H. Daughaday

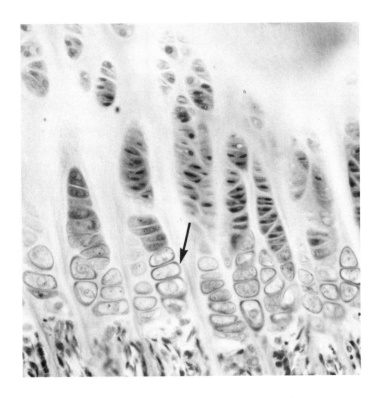

Figure 15. Growth plate cartilage in a bone.
Arrow points to cartilage cells that have enlarged
under the influence of growth hormone IGF.

in St. Louis, decided to try to duplicate it using cartilage cells cultured in a broth in a dish. They applied GH to the culture and waited. Then, something remarkable occurred.

Nothing happened.

The cultured cartilage stubbornly refused to respond to GH, in spite of the fact that cartilage in the body had a well-known, and dramatic, response. What was wrong?

Instead of throwing the culture out and forgetting about their puzzling results, Daughaday and Salmon concluded that GH must act by stimulating the production of *another* hormone in the body, which is then carried by the bloodstream to cartilage to cause growth. And, by testing fractions of blood serum from animals treated with growth hormone, they were able to show that GH does indeed cause the production of a hormone from the liver that *is* able to directly stimulate the growth of cartilage in culture. This secondary hormone, which they called somatomedin but which is now recognized as belonging to a family of hormones called *insulinlike growth factors* (IGFs), has a powerful influence upon the growth of many tissues, as well as that of cartilage.

As it turns out, insulinlike growth factors are now allowing us to have a better understanding of some of the actions of estrogen. You may recall that estrogen causes women to have a shorter stature than men. This now appears partly due to an interference with the action of IGFs upon cartilage. In the uterus, on the other hand, estrogen appears to *enhance* the actions of IGFs, causing enlargement of the uterus and the multiplication of some uterine cells. This is only one example in endocrinology of how the *interaction* of two or more hormones, often in complicated ways, provides the explanation for a given biological effect. The details of why estrogen would interfere with IGFs in the bones and yet reinforce IGFs in the uterus are still unknown.

The discovery of IGFs also has helped us to understand how overall growth can be controlled. How do the brain and pituitary keep track of how big our bodies are so that the amount of GH can be properly regulated? In actual fact, the pituitary does not need some sort of mysterious measuring device that monitors the growth of the body; instead, the blood level of IGF is itself monitored by the pituitary so that GH is not secreted in excessive amounts. This self-regulating process of negative feedback, which was long known to control pituitary basophil activity, now is thus recognized to also apply to acidophil cells that secrete GH.

What happens if this control process of negative feedback fails, so that too much GH or IGF is secreted? The results depend upon at what age this failure begins. If a failure in this control process begins before puberty, at a time when epiphyseal cartilage is still growing, then excessive bone growth occurs that can lead to gigantism and heights of 8 feet or more. Failure of growth regulation at later ages, when the epiphyseal plates are inactive or "closed," can only produce overgrowth of other soft tissues, resulting in acromegaly. Most of us reach a level of growth, caused by GH and IGF, that appears strongly regulated by as yet unidentified genes that we inherit from our parents.

A number of curiosities were uncovered along the road to understanding how GH works. Insulinlike growth factors, for example, appear to affect the development of many tissues in embryos. For example, Dr. David Beebe in Bethesda, Maryland, has found that an IGF is responsible for the transformation of developing eye cells into extremely long, transparent lens fibers that make up the structure of the lens of the eye. Continued study of IGFs should reveal more fascinating aspects of their role in cell growth, as in cancer (see below).

PROLACTIN

A second type of pituitary acidophil cell secretes a hormone called *prolactin*, which is a protein hormone that shares some of the chemical and biological properties of GH. While both men and women possess this hormone, a definite biological role for prolactin has been firmly established only in women: prolactin stimulates glandular tissue in the breasts to produce milk.

CONTROL OF THE ANTERIOR PITUITARY

The fact that the brain is physically connected to the pituitary and that the brain directs the pituitary to release hormones such as ACTH during stressful situations long suggested that the brain somehow exerts some kind of control over the anterior pituitary. A detailed understanding of this control, however, proved elusive for some time. Did nerves from the hypothalamus control the pituitary, or was some other mechanism responsible? One of the first people to provide an answer to this question was the English endocrinologist Geoffrey Harris.

Harris, in 1950, determined that cutting the stalk connecting the pituitary to the median eminence of the hypothalamus caused the pituitary of a rat to stop secreting for a while. After several weeks, however, the pituitary started working again! Harris found that this was due to regeneration of tiny blood vessels that connected the pituitary to the brain; when he inserted a small piece of wax into the cut stalk to prevent the blood vessels from growing together again, the blockade of anterior pituitary function was permanent. These and other experiments made it clear that some chemicals must be secreted into blood vessels from hypothalamic nerve cells, and that these chemicals are carried down the vessels to the anterior pituitary to control its function. What were these chemicals?

RELEASING HORMONES—COMMAND SIGNALS FROM THE BRAIN TO THE PITUITARY

One of the most dramatic stories in modern endocrinology is that of the race between two teams of scientists—one headed by Andrew Schally in New Orleans, and the other by Roger Guillemin in California—to discover what these chemicals were. The task, as it turned out, was difficult. The hypothalamic chemicals these teams sought proved to be present in very tiny amounts, making recovery of the chemical from the hypothalamus very difficult. Roger Guillemin, for example, went to meat-packing plants to obtain hypothalami from slaughtered sheep. He and his team obtained hypothalami from 5 million sheep brains, collecting brain fragments amounting to 50 tons of hypothalamic tissue! After laborious extraction and testing of fractions of 300,000 of these fragments, 1 *milligram* of a pure chemical was finally obtained. This first hypothalamic chemical, called **thyrotropin-releasing hormone** (TRH) because it stimulated the release of TSH from the pituitary, proved to be a small protein composed of a chain of only three amino acids.

Every few years during the 1970s, the teams of Guillemin or Schally (Schally had obtained hypothalami from pigs) would examine yet another batch of test tubes containing hypothalamic extracts and would work to discover yet another hypothalamic releasing hormone. By 1977, Guillemin and Schally were jointly awarded the Nobel Prize for their work. At the present time, quite a few hypothalamic hormones have been identified. Four of these are called releasing hormones (RH), since they stimulate the release of hormones from the anterior pituitary: LH-RH, TRH, GH-RH, and CRH (this one releases the ACTH-endorphin-MSH precursor from basophils). Other substances secreted from hypothalamic neurons, such as a chemical called **dopamine** and another protein called **somatostatin** (so-mat-o-STAT-in) have an *inhibitory* influence upon the secretion of prolactin and growth hormone respectively. There is some indirect evidence for the existence of chemicals that stimulate the release of only prolactin and FSH, but the identity of these substances is still unknown.

The discovery of these hypothalamic hormones has been very useful. It is now known that they are not only present in the hypothalamus but also in other nerve cells throughout the brain, which secrete them from nerve endings as so-called neurotransmitters to affect the function of neighboring nerve cells. For example, motor neurons in the spinal cord use TRH as a neurotransmitter, while other neurons in the sympathetic nervous system use LH-RH. It appears that these chemicals originated as common neurotransmitters and are used by hypothalamic neurons only for the specialized task of controlling the pituitary. This is not all: more recently, it has become clear that some nerve cells even use hormones found in the pituitary, like endorphin, prolactin, or LH, as neurotransmitters. Thus, the distinction between the nervous system and endocrine system has gotten very blurry in recent times, a fact that reminds us that nerve cells and endocrine cells are very closely related in both function and development.

Now that releasing hormones, and the specific nerve cells that make them, are understood, it will eventually become possible to understand the connections between nerve cells in the brain that control hormone release and phenomena like puberty, stress-induced release of ACTH, the influence of the time of the day on hormone secretion, etc. The branch of endocrinology devoted to problems such as this has become known as **neuroendocrinology**.

POSTERIOR PITUITARY HORMONES— VASOPRESSIN AND OXYTOCIN

Although the posterior pituitary is composed mainly of nerve fibers and the cells that support and nourish them, it too is capable of producing hormones. One of the earliest proofs that this is so came from a report by a German endocrinologist, Alfred Frank. Frank in 1908 examined a patient who had been shot in the head and had mainly recovered. His principal complaint was that he was excessively thirsty and drank and urinated much more than normal. Frank took X rays of the man's head and found that the bullet had lodged near the posterior pituitary, damaging it! He concluded from this that the posterior lobe must produce a hormone that affects water balance in the body.

Further study of the posterior pituitary showed that it did indeed secrete a hormone that influenced water metabolism, and that the hormone was probably manufactured in hypothalamic neurons and transported down nerve fibers into the posterior lobe. Once the hormone arrived there, it accumulated in large, dark-staining swellings at nerve endings that were first described in 1908 by the English physiologist Percy Herring. These accumulations of hormone, now called **Herring bodies**, are shown in Figure 16. They can be of many shapes and sizes, but they all function as temporary storage depots of hormones until a need arises for secretion into the bloodstream.

The hormone that Frank postulated is now known to be a small protein, only nine amino acids long, called *vasopressin*. Vasopressin acts on the kidney to enable it to produce small amounts of concentrated urine. Without vasopressin, the kidney produces large amounts of dilute urine, leading to a great deal of water loss from the body. Rare cases of posterior pituitary damage thus cause excessive urination, a condition called diabetes insipidus, and an accompanying powerful thirst.

Herring bodies not only contain vasopressin, but also another hormone that is similar in amino acid composition to vasopressin. This hormone, called **oxytocin**, is important for the delivery and nourishment of a baby. Oxytocin causes a certain type of muscle called smooth muscle to contract. When smooth muscle in the uterus responds to oxytocin, the uterine contractions during labor are strengthened, enabling a baby to be born. This hormonal effect, in fact, can be taken advantage of when labor is progressing too slowly: by giving an artificial form of oxytocin intravenously, labor can be speeded up so that a mother doesn't become exhausted. Later, after the baby is born, oxytocin acts upon the smooth muscle surrounding the glandular tissue in the breasts, causing expulsion of milk toward the nipple.

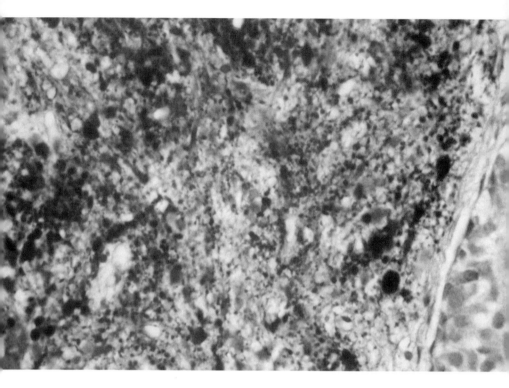

Figure 16. Posterior pituitary. Dark droplets
are hormone-containing Herring bodies.

Both of these hormones are made in two large, dark-staining collections of nerve cells in the hypothalamus called the supraoptic and paraventricular (PV) nuclei (Figure 17). Nerve cells in both nuclei make one or the other posterior pituitary hormone and transport it down nerve fibers that terminate in the posterior lobe.

These hypothalamic nuclei are remarkable in several ways. First, they contain a higher density of capillaries than any other tissue in the brain. This extraordinary number of capillaries is doubtless related to one of their

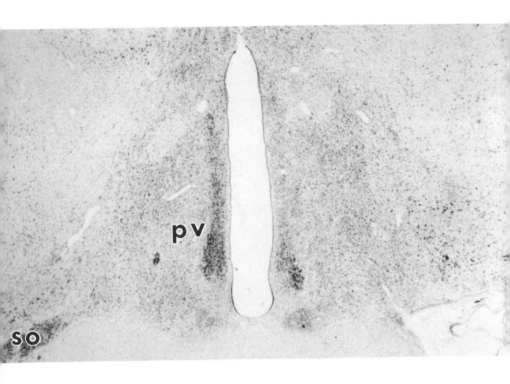

Figure 17. Sites of origin of posterior pituitary hormones in the monkey hypothalamus. Nerve cells in two separate clusters, called nuclei, make these hormones. The supraoptic nuclei (so) are positioned superior to the optic tracts and the paraventricular nuclei (pv) lie next to a midline, fluid-filled cavity called the third ventricle.

functions: vasopressin-containing neurons appear to constantly "sample" the bloodstream to measure how much sodium is in it. If the blood begins to become too salty, the neurons react by releasing vasopressin, which instructs the kidney to conserve body water.

Another unusual feature of the paraventricular

nucleus in particular is that it controls a great variety of hormonal functions. In addition to vasopressin-containing neurons, the PV nucleus also contains neurons that make TRH and CRH, and so can regulate the anterior lobe as well as the posterior lobe of the pituitary. Also, the PV nucleus sends instructions to the sympathetic nervous system and the adrenal medulla to activate these tissues during stress. Clearly, this collection of neurons is one of the "busiest" in the hypothalamus and regulates a wide variety of functions.

S I X

HOW HORMONES WORK

As we have seen, hormones have an amazing number of powerful effects upon the body. Depending upon the state of the endocrine system, a person can become thin or fat, acquire many different sex-specific features, have a rapid or slow metabolism, feel pain or be insensitive to it, and grow to the height of a giant or only to that of a dwarf. Because these effects are so varied, each action of a hormone undoubtedly is somewhat unique for each type of cell affected or for each part of the body. In spite of this, many details of how hormones produce some of these amazing effects are now becoming known.

Most of the hormones we have discussed in the preceding chapters are *protein* hormones, made up of long chains of simple molecules called amino acids. These hormones include insulin, glucagon, parathyroid hormone, calcitonin, IGFs, and all of the pituitary hormones. The remaining hormones—sex hormones and hormones of the adrenal cortex—are *steroid* hormones that are chemically quite different. These hormones are slightly different forms of the cholesterol molecule and fall into the same category of substances as fats or oils (lipids). These two types of hormones each have characteristic mechanisms of changing cell function.

PROTEIN HORMONES

Most protein hormones are long chains of amino acids typically between 50 to 100 amino acids long. The exact sequence of amino acids for each hormone has been worked out within the last five to ten years. This amino acid sequence, different for each protein hormone, causes a completed protein chain to fold up to form a tiny object with a three-dimensional shape specific for that particular sequence of amino acids. Exactly how the differing chemical properties of varying sequences of amino acids interact to cause this specific three-dimensional shape is still a basic and unsolved problem in biology.

What *is* known at this point is that each protein hormone takes on its own particular shape after being manufactured and secreted by an endocrine cell. Because of this, a hormone can attach to other protein molecules, called **receptor proteins**, that are present on the surface of target cells. All the powerful effects of protein hormones can come about without the hormone ever entering a cell: protein hormones need only to lightly stick to the surface of a cell to have their effects.

As outlined in Figure 18, receptor proteins for hormones float in the thin film of oil (lipid) that forms a watertight barrier around each cell in the body. This film of lipid is called the **cell membrane**. It is not unusual for a single cell to have 10,000 to 100,000 hormone receptor proteins scattered about on its cell membrane. Each receptor protein can bind (attach to) a hormone because it has a shape that is complementary to the hormone; that is, the hormone and the receptor fit together like two pieces of a jigsaw puzzle.

Once a hormone binds to its cell receptor, one or

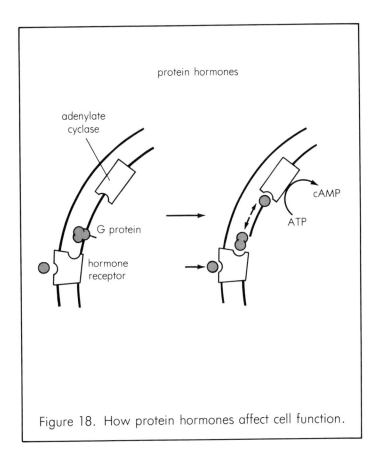

protein hormones

adenylate
cyclase

cAMP

ATP

G protein

hormone
receptor

Figure 18. How protein hormones affect cell function.

more intracellular substances, called **second messengers**, are formed to carry out the instructions the hormone is giving to the cell.

Figure 18 shows one common pathway by which protein hormones affect cells. When a protein hormone binds to its receptor, the receptor reacts by changing its shape. This allows it to interact with other proteins that float around on the surface of a cell. One of these is called a **G protein**, after its ability to bind a small molecule called GTP (guanosine triphosphate). G proteins have very important effects upon the function of a cell.

81

When a hormone receptor binds a protein hormone, it alters its shape and attaches to a G protein.

The G protein responds by splitting into two parts. One of the parts remains attached to the hormone receptor, while the other part floats away and attaches to yet another protein.

This third protein is an enzyme called **adenylate cyclase** (a-DEN-i-late SI-klase), which responds to the G protein fragment by transforming a molecule called ATP (adenosine triphosphate) into a small molecule called cyclic AMP (cAMP). It is this small molecule that acts as a powerful second messenger in the cell. Since thousands of molecules of cAMP can be generated each time a hormone binds to a receptor, only tiny amounts of hormone can have a greatly amplified effect upon a cell. This amplifying property of this whole series of events is probably why such a complicated mechanism was evolved in the first place. The final result is that a protein hormone can cause drastic changes in proteins that control cell shape and cell metabolism.

Although these steps look complicated, they actually require a very short time to take place. As a matter of fact, within two to five minutes after injecting a hormone into the bloodstream, dramatic hormonal effects upon cell function can be detected. Conversely, if a hormone detaches from a receptor, its effects disappear within an equally short time.

While many hormones use this pathway to affect cells, some hormones have slightly different modes of action. For example, some hormone-activated G proteins don't cause the release of cAMP, but instead cause the production of small lipid molecules that themselves act as second messengers.

STEROID HORMONES

Steroid hormones have a structure that is very different from that of protein hormones, and act upon cells in an

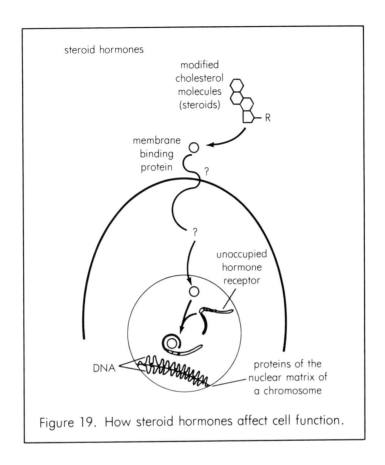

steroid hormones

modified
cholesterol
molecules
(steroids)

R

membrane
binding
protein

?

?

unoccupied
hormone
receptor

DNA

proteins of the
nuclear matrix of
a chromosome

Figure 19. How steroid hormones affect cell function.

equally different way. Steroids like adrenal cortical hormones and sex hormones are made from molecules of cholesterol. Various smaller molecules (abbreviated as R in Figure 19) are added to this cholesterol to produce specific types of steroid hormones. Since cholesterol (and steroid hormones) are lipidlike molecules, they dissolve in oils rather than in water and have different chemical properties than protein hormones. As a matter of fact, many steroid hormones can be injected into an animal only by dissolving them in oils like peanut oil or other vegetable oils.

83

Since they are so poorly soluble in water, steroid hormones are transported throughout the bloodstream by "carrier" proteins that loosely attach to them. Once a steroid hormone arrives at a cell, it appears to have the ability to pass right through the cell membrane and enter the cytoplasm, perhaps by associating with other proteins that are not well understood yet. Unlike protein hormones, steroid hormones must enter a cell and be transported to the cell nucleus to affect cell function. This is another key difference between steroid and protein hormones.

Once inside the cell, steroids also bind to receptor proteins, with the difference that these receptor proteins are found floating within the cell nucleus. When a steroid receptor protein binds to a hormone, it also changes its shape. Thus, the first step in changing cell function taken by both steroid hormones and protein hormones is to bind to a receptor protein and thereby change the shape of that protein.

When a steroid receptor protein changes its shape, it is then able to bind to DNA, the genetic material in chromosomes that dictates the functions of each of our cells. In Figure 19, loops of DNA belonging to a single chromosome are shown attached to a "rope" of proteins connected to the nuclear membrane. These proteins, called nuclear matrix proteins, are thought to form the "core" of each chromosome and may help steroid hormone receptors attach to DNA.

When steroid receptors bind to DNA, they attach to specific sites on the DNA and "stick up" from it like flags. This causes other nuclear proteins to settle down on the DNA nearby and start "reading" the message on a nearby gene. This message may, for example, tell the cell to start accumulating fat, as in estrogen-stimulated fat cells beneath the skin of a woman.

All of these steps, unlike the ones activated by protein hormones, are time-consuming. As a matter of fact, changes in cell function take as long as four to six hours to develop after injection of a steroid hormone. This disadvantage is offset by the fact that steroid-induced changes in function are likely to persist far longer than effects of protein hormones.

THYROID HORMONE

The way thyroxine acts upon cells long was regarded as something of a mystery. Thyroxine is too small a molecule to act like a protein and does not bind to receptors on cell surfaces. On the other hand, it is chemically unlike steroids, so for a long while it was hard to decide how it influences cells. Now, however, it has become clear that thyroxine attaches to proteins that are very like steroid receptors, with the difference that they bind thyroxine and not steroids. Thyroxine, then, also appears to mainly influence cells via an action upon DNA.

HORMONES AND CANCER

It has long been known that some of the features of cancer cells resemble features of cells exposed to hormones. For example, cells in tumors grow and multiply rapidly, crowding out normal cells and robbing the rest of the body of nutrients. Cells exposed to hormones also can grow rapidly, although they don't have the wild, uncontrolled growth of tumors. Also, some organs that are sensitive to steroid hormones, such as the breasts, the prostate gland, and the testes, tend to become cancerous more frequently and have tumors that may require steroid hormones to grow. We now know that these shared properties of cancerous and hormone-induced growth are not simply coincidences.

Research over the last ten years has identified genes in the DNA that appear to cause cells to become cancerous. These genes have been given abbreviated names by molecular biologists: src, for example, is found in sarcoma-type tumors, whereas other cancer-causing genes like ras, raf, erb, myc, fos, and jun were identified in other types of cancer. These genes apparently cause the production of proteins that regulate cell growth in a variety of ways. Some of these genes are also activated by hormones to increase cell growth. Insulin and IGFs, for example, apparently cause certain muscle cells to grow by activating the myc gene. Other cancer-causing genes apparently produce hormone receptor proteins that are permanently activated even if no hormone is present, leading to uncontrolled cell growth. Still other cancer-producing genes, like erb, resemble steroid hormone receptors and bind to DNA to cause uncontrolled cell growth. While an understanding of these relationships between cancerous and hormone-induced changes in cell function is still in the early stages, there is much reason for optimism that the molecular mechanisms underlying these changes will become known reasonably soon.

GLOSSARY

acidophils. Pituitary cells stained intensely by dyes with acid characteristics. These cells secrete prolactin or growth hormone.

adenylate cyclase. An enzyme, bound to the membrane of target cells, that generates a small molecule called cyclic AMP. When adenylate cyclase is activated by hormones binding to the cell membrane, it sends cAMP into the cell as a "message" that cell function should be altered.

adrenal glands. Small glands located just above the kidneys that produce steroid hormones and norepinephrine.

adrenocorticotrophic hormone (ACTH). Hormone produced by the pituitary gland that stimulates the function of the adrenal cortex.

aldosterone. One of the steroid hormones secreted by the adrenal glands. This hormone causes the body to conserve sodium.

amino acid. One of twenty-three naturally occurring compounds in the body that all contain an acid molecule (COOH) on one end and an amino molecule (NH_2) on the other end. Amino acids can be linked together to form long chains called proteins.

androgens. Sex hormones similar to testosterone that have a masculinizing effect upon the body.

antibodies. Small protein molecules, produced by cells of the immune system, that attach to foreign substances that do not belong in the body and which help destroy these foreign substances.

87

basophils. Pituitary cells stained intensely by dyes that have the features of a "base" rather than an acid. These cells secrete luteinizing hormone, follicle stimulating hormone, or thyroid stimulating hormone.

blood-brain barrier. An unusual feature of brain blood vessels that prevents many substances, including protein hormones, from entering nervous tissue in most areas of the brain.

calcitonin. Hormone produced by the thyroid gland that lowers blood levels of calcium by increasing the storage of calcium in bones.

cancer. Disease in which an uncontrolled growth of some cells in the body leads to the creation of cell masses called tumors. Cancer can lead to general weakness and death.

cell. The smallest unit of independent life.

cell membrane. A watertight film of oil (lipid) and protein that encloses all cells.

chromosomes. Long molecules of DNA, found in the cell nucleus, that contain the genetic information needed to operate cells.

corpus luteum. A specialized region of ovarian tissue, formed from cells that once had surrounded an oocyte, that secretes progesterone in the latter half of the menstrual cycle.

cortisol. A steroid hormone, secreted by the adrenal glands, that elevates blood levels of glucose and which reduces inflammation in damaged tissues or in arthritis.

cytoplasm. Watery material between the cell nucleus and the cell membrane that contains the cell's nutrients and cell structures.

diabetes mellitus. Disease with symptoms of high levels of sugar in the blood and excessive thirst and urination. Caused by an insufficient action of insulin.

DNA. Deoxyribonucleic acid, a long molecule composed of sequences of four compounds that are arranged in a sequence that "spells out" information, written in a genetic "code," that guides cell function.

dopamine. A chemical secreted by some nerve cells to stimulate and "talk to" neighboring nerve cells; may be used by hypothalamic nerve cells to inhibit the secretion of prolactin.

endocrine gland. A gland that secretes something directly into the bloodstream to affect the function of other organs.

endorphin. A protein produced by pituitary cells that can act as the body's "endogenous morphine" and reduce the perception of pain.

enzyme. A protein that speeds up the chemical transformation of molecules.

epinephrine. A hormone secreted by the adrenal medulla that can make the heart beat faster and which can change blood pressure.

epiphyseal plate. A specialized layer of cartilage present near the ends of some bones that widens under the influence of growth hormones and which causes bones to lengthen.

estrogen. A female sex hormone, produced by the ovaries.

follicle-stimulating hormone. A hormone secreted by the pituitary that causes sperm maturation in men and oocyte maturation in women.

G protein. A small protein in the cell membrane that can interact with a hormone receptor protein nearby if a hormone is present. When G proteins interact with a hormone-hormone receptor complex, another important membrane protein, adenylate cyclase, is activated to affect cell function.

gene. Portion of DNA on a chromosome containing the information needed to make one protein. Abnormal genes, when inherited, result in abnormal proteins and an abnormal function of affected cells.

glucagon. A hormone secreted by the pancreas that can lower levels of blood sugar.

glucocorticoid. a type of adrenal hormone (e.g., cortisol), that raises levels of blood sugar.

glucose. A type of sugar resulting from the digestion of many foods. Used as a major source of energy for many cells.

goiter. An enlarged thyroid gland. This enlargement can be due to overactivity (toxic goiter) or to under-activity (simple goiter).

granulosa cells. One of the two types of cells that surround maturing oocytes in the ovary.

herring bodies. Accumulations of vasopressin and oxytocin in swollen nerve endings found in the posterior pituitary gland.

hormone. A molecule carried throughout the bloodstream that affects cell function.

hypothalamus. Plural: *hypothalami.* A small area on the underside of the brain that controls the secretion of pituitary hormones and which regulates appetite, reproduction, and body temperature.

insulin. A hormone secreted by the pancreas that lowers blood sugar.

insulin-like growth factor. A hormone with some similarities in structure to insulin, but which mainly stimulates the growth of bones and other tissues.

islets of langerhans. Small, spherical collections of endocrine cells scattered throughout the pancreas.

leydig cells. Cells in the testes that produce the male sex hormone, testosterone.

luteinizing hormone. A hormone secreted by the pituitary gland that causes testosterone production in men and ovulation and estrogen production in women.

melanocyte-stimulating hormone. Hormone secreted by the pituitary that increases the production of melanin in pigmented cells of the skin.

menopause. Age at which menstrual cycles, ovulation, and reproductive ability in women ceases.

menstruation. Period in a woman's monthly reproductive cycle in which cells and blood are shed from the lining of the uterus.

monocytes. Cells originating in bone marrow that can fuse together to form osteoclasts.

negative feedback. A mechanism for the control of hormone secretion. For example, when the thyroid gland makes thyroxine, the thyroxine inhibits (by negative feedback) the secretion of thyroid-stimulating hormone by the pituitary.

oocytes. Maturing egg cells found in the ovary.

osmosis. The tendency for water to pass through a permeable membrane from a dilute solution of a chemical to a concentrated solution of a chemical.

osteoclasts. Cells that settle down on the surface of a bone and dissolve bone tissue to release calcium into the circulation. Stimulated by parathyroid hormone.

ovulation. Release of a fully mature oocyte from the ovary. Occurs once a month, under the influence of a rapid rise in blood levels of FSH and LH.

oxytocin. Small protein hormone secreted by the posterior pituitary that can stimulate labor or milk release by acting upon specialized muscle in the uterus or mammary glands.

pancreas. A gland located beneath the stomach that produces digestive juices and hormones.

parafollicular cells. Cells adjacent to thyroid follicles that produce calcitonin, a hormone that lowers blood concentrations of calcium.

parathyroid hormone. Hormone produced by the parathyroid glands that increases blood concentrations of calcium.

pituitary gland. Gland suspended from the base of the brain. It secretes hormones that control other endocrine glands.

placebo effect. Psychological benefit occurring when a patient takes an inactive drug that he believes is actually helpful medication.

progesterone. A steroid hormone produced by the corpus luteum that prepares the uterus for pregnancy.

prolactin. Protein hormone produced by the pituitary gland that stimulates the synthesis of milk in mammary glands.

pro-opiomelanocortin. Long protein molecule produced by pituitary cells that is broken up into fragments that become ACTH, melanocyte-stimulating hormone, and endorphin.

protein. A long molecule composed of many amino acids joined together. Each protein has a specific shape and function.

puberty. The time at which sex organs begin to develop.

somatostatin. Small protein produced by hypothalamic nerve cells that inhibits growth hormone secretion by the pituitary.

somatotropin. Another term for the pituitary hormone, growth hormone.

steroid hormones. Lipid soluble hormones manufactured from the cholesterol molecule. Produced by the adrenal gland, ovaries, and testes.

tetany. Muscle spasms resulting from a drastic fall in blood concentrations of calcium. Can be caused by parathyroid removal.

theca cells. Cells in the ovary that surround a developing oocyte and which secrete estrogen.

thyroglobulin. Large protein produced by thyroid cells. Iodine is added to it, and iodine-rich fragments of it are cleaved from the protein to produce thyroxine.

thyroid gland. Endocrine gland wrapped around the trachea that produces thyroxine and calcitonin.

thyroid-stimulating hormone. Pituitary hormone that increases the activity of the thyroid gland.

thyroxine. Thyroid hormone that stimulates metabolic rate.

vasopressin. Small hormone produced by the posterior lobe of the pituitary that increases blood pressure and causes the production of concentrated urine by the kidney.

FOR FURTHER READING

Bennett, W. *The Dieter's Dilemma: Eating Less and Weighing More.* New York: Basic Books, 1982.

Guyton, A. C. *Textbook of Medical Physiology.* 7th ed. Philadelphia: W. B. Saunders, 1986.

Krieger, D. T. and J. T. Hughes, Eds. *Neuroendocrinology.* New York: H. P. Publishing, 1980.

Medvei, V. C. *A History of Endocrinology.* Boston: MTP Press, 1982.

Nourse, Alan. *Hormones.* New York: Franklin Watts, 1979.

Young, John K. *Cells: Amazing Forms and Functions.* New York: Franklin Watts, 1990.

INDEX

Italicized page numbers refer to illustrations.